YIN YANG RESET

TARA AKUNA R.AC.
SARA WARD R.AC.
with Marial Shea

Yin Yang Reset

Copyright © 2023 Sara Ward and Tara Akuna

All rights reserved. No part of this publication may be reproduced, stored in a retrieval system, or transmitted in any form or by any means, electronic, mechanical, photocopying, recording or otherwise, without the prior permission of the author or publisher.

This book is sold subject to the condition that is shall not, by way of trade or otherwise, be lent, re-sold, hired out or otherwise circulated without the author's or publisher's prior consent in any form binding or cover other than that in which it is published and without a similar condition including this condition being imposed on the subsequent purchaser.

Book design by Michael Boalch
Cover design by Verity Casey

Disclaimer

The material appearing in this book is provided for informational purposes only. It should not be used as a substitute for professional medical advice, diagnosis, or treatment. Always consult your professional healthcare providers before beginning any new treatment. It is your responsibility to research the accuracy, completeness, and usefulness of all opinions and other information found in this book.

Yin Yang Reset and YINYANGDIETS.COM assume no responsibility or liability for any consequence resulting directly or indirectly from any action or inaction you take based on the information found in this book. Your use of this book indicates your agreement to these terms.

To our children, for testing our recipes and giving us uncensored, honest feedback.

To our husbands, for being our rocks, cheerleaders, voices of reason, and eater of all things.

To our patients, for urging us to simplify and update Traditional Chinese Medicine so we can ALL take charge of our health. Thank you for allowing us to be part of your journey.

And to you, our readers, for welcoming us into your kitchens.

Contents

Introducing Sara, Tara, and Yin Yang Reset   11

Part I The Yin Yang Reset User's Manual 15

    Why Does Yin Yang Reset Work Where Other Diets Fail?   16

    Introducing Food Formulas   16

    Finding Your Reset with the QUIZ   18

    Help, My Quiz Results Are Not Clear!   26

    Boost Your Reset with Movement, Hydration, Skin Brushing, and Sleep   27

    Why and How to Get Off Coffee   36

    Foods to Avoid for All Resets   38

    How Each Reset Rolls Out   40

    Three Lists to Simplify Your Food Therapy   41

    The Meal Plans and Recipes   42

    Give Yourself the Gift of a Bite-Sized Reset   44

    Yin Yang Reset Is Here When You Need It   45

    Rinse and Repeat   45

    Are You Getting Enough Protein?   46

    Hot Smoothies? Are You Kidding?   49

Part II The Resets & Recipes — 51

Blood Deficiency Reset — 53

What's Happening in Your Body When Your Blood Is Deficient? — 53

What Deficient Blood can look like — 54

Goals for Building Blood — 55

Kitchen Medicine for Building Blood — 56

Activities for Building Blood — 58

Beverages for Building Blood — 60

How to Make Medicinal Teas — 61

Blood Deficiency Reset Food Chart — 62

Sample Blood-Building Meal Plans — 64

Blood-Building Breakfasts — 67

Blood-Building Lunches — 75

Blood-Building Dinners — 85

Blood-Building Desserts — 99

Dampness Reset — 105

What's Happening in Your Body with Dampness? — 105

What Dampness can look like — 107

Goals for Draining Dampness — 108

Kitchen Medicine for Draining Dampness — 109

A Word of Warning about Damp-Draining Foods	111
Getting Started with the Dampness Reset	113
Activities for Draining Dampness	114
Beverages for Draining Dampness	115
Dampness Reset Food Chart	116
Sample Damp-Draining Meal Plans	118
Damp-Draining Breakfasts	121
Damp-Draining Lunches	131
Damp-Draining Dinners	143
Damp-Draining Desserts	157

Qi Deficiency Reset — 163

What's Happening in Your Body when Your Qi Is Deficient?	163
What Qi Deficiency can look like	164
Goals for Building Qi	165
Kitchen Medicine for Building Qi	167
Getting Started with Building Qi	169
Activities for Building Qi	170
Beverages for Building Qi	172
Qi Deficiency Reset Food Chart	174
Sample Qi-Building Meal Plans	176

Qi-Building Breakfasts	179
Qi-Building Lunches	189
Qi-Building Dinners	199
Qi-Building Desserts	217

Qi Stagnation Reset — 223

What's Happening in Your Body when You Have Qi Stagnation?	223
What Qi Stagnation can look like	225
Goals for Moving Qi	226
Kitchen Medicine for Moving Qi	227
Getting Started with Moving Qi	228
Activities for Moving Qi	229
Beverages that Move Qi	231
Qi Stagnation Reset Food Chart	232
Sample Qi-Moving Meal Plans	234
Qi Stagnation Breakfasts	237
Qi Stagnation Lunches	247
Qi Stagnation Dinners	257
Qi Stagnation Desserts	277

Yin Deficiency Reset   **283**

    What's Happening in Your Body when Your Yin Is Deficient?   283

    What Yin Deficiency can look like   285

    Goals for Building Yin   286

    Kitchen Medicine for Building Yin   287

    Getting Started with building Yin   289

    Activities for Building Yin   290

    Beverages for Building Yin   292

    Yin Deficiency Reset Food Chart   294

    Sample Yin-Building Meal Plans   296

    Yin-Building Breakfasts   299

    Yin-Building Lunches   307

    Yin-Building Dinners   317

    Yin-Building Desserts   333

Frequently Asked Questions   **339**

Acknowledgments   **347**

About the Authors   **351**

Introducing Sara, Tara, and Yin Yang Reset

Welcome to Yin Yang Reset! We're so glad you've showed up for yourself. Whether you're living with a serious chronic illness or you're simply running on empty, Yin Yang Reset is a short-term program designed to reboot your vital energy and restore your zest for life.

We are acupuncturists Sara and Tara, and we've spent years witnessing the amazing healing power of Traditional Chinese Medicine (TCM) in our clinical practices. Every day, we get to help people heal from all kinds of acute and chronic conditions. We love our patients, and we never want to stop doing acupuncture.

But what about people who can't get in to our clinics? What about folks who can't afford acupuncture? And what about our own patients when they're between visits? Or, what if – here's a crazy thought – what if there was a pandemic, and *nobody* could come into the clinic!

So, we asked ourselves: How can we put the super-effective healing wisdom of TCM into the hands of ... well, *every*body?

We looked at our own lives and asked, how do we heal ourselves and our families? We realized it's the food, hands down. We've seen Chinese food therapy work wonders both at home and in the clinic. Food is our medicine. It's the rock-solid foundation of our well-being, each and every day.

But, after slogging through confusing Traditional Chinese Medicine texts and boring food lists, we wondered: does tapping into ancient wisdom have to be so damn complicated?

We didn't think so. As rebellious acupuncturists, we decided to shake up our industry by going DIY with TCM. So, we rolled up our sleeves and created Yin Yang Reset, our 21st-century update of ancient Chinese food therapy designed to bring an imbalanced body back into balance. We created a simple diagnostic quiz and five DIY programs that use short-term food therapy you can easily apply in your very own kitchen, using everyday ingredients. Our goal was to get you up dancing again.

What do we mean by "short-term food therapy"? This program will bring you quickly back into balance. It's all about turning your gut-brain connection back on and drastically reducing – even eliminating – your symptoms. Most people see results within two to four weeks. Some with more stubborn symptoms stay on their Reset for up to three months. We'll explain more about this as we go.

We called this program Yin Yang Reset because yin and yang are the complementary forces of nature at the core of Traditional Chinese Medicine (TCM). Very simply, yang is active, light, and warm; it brings change. Yin is quiet, dark, and cool; it maintains stability. Yin and yang are constantly balancing and depending upon each other all through nature, including in your body. And one of the fastest ways to bring yin and yang back into balance is by using food as medicine.

We LOVE food, so we knew right from the get-go that Yin Yang Reset would have to include recipes that taste flat-out freakin' DELICIOUS. So, not only have the recipes been tested by us, they've won the coveted seal of approval from friends, family, patients, and tiny, picky children.

Each of the five Resets is flexible. Can't find an ingredient? Want to retrofit a favourite recipe using the Yin-Yang principles? No problem, we'll show you how to be a creative kitchen ninja. Once you understand the basics of your Reset, you'll know how to swap out unhelpful ingredients for healing foods that will rebalance your body.

Is your Reset a forever diet? Heck, no. The essence of yin and yang is dynamic change. This means the Reset that works for you today might not work next year, or even next month. This is short-term food therapy for your beautiful bod as it is right now. That's what the quiz is for, to find out where you're at NOW and what you need to rebalance.

As busy working moms, we knew the Resets would have to be EASY. That's why we've provided a handy food chart and meal plans to make the whole process doable. No need to hunt down weird ingredients. A trip to your local grocery store or farmer's market, and you're ready to roll.

And speaking of shopping, we've got great news if you've been forking out a fortune in the "health care" aisle. You'll experience these positive changes without the expense (and possible adverse effects) of high-dose supplements and gimmicky processed "superfoods."

Yin Yang Reset is your toolkit for self-transformation. It's not just a product we're flogging. It's how we feed our own families and live our lives. Now, we're offering you these tools so you can take control of *your* healing. We want to get you feeling great again, or maybe even for the first time.

Simple, accessible, affordable, and tailored to your specific health pattern, Yin Yang Reset is ready to use right out of the box. And, we promise, no esoteric terms, back bends, or mind-numbing concepts. Just kitchen medicine for EVERY body.

Okay, let's get started. If you have any questions along the way, visit our website YINYANGDIETS.COM.

Part I
The Yin Yang Reset User's Manual

Why Does Yin Yang Reset Work Where Other Diets Fail?

If you're like most of our patients — and us! — you've probably tried a LOT of diets and protocols in an effort to be well. Enough, already. Here's why Yin Yang Reset is in a league of its own.

First, it's not a food fad. Yin Yang Reset is based on traditional Chinese food therapy, which has been tested and refined over thousands of years.

Second, it's not one-size-fits-all. Yin Yang Reset is tailored to your specific constitution at this moment in time. It's a flexible treatment PLAN, not a diet, and it gives you solid takeaways you can immediately — and easily — put into action.

And third, even though Yin Yang Reset is short-term food therapy, we bet it'll get you into a healthier groove for life. Here's the deal: follow your Reset for two weeks, or up to three months, max. Then try — just try — to go back to how you were eating before. Go ahead, we dare you to stop eating all those delicious Yin Yang Reset foods that curbed your symptoms and restored your energy. We've seen it happen time and again: once people understand how to use food to feel better, there's no going back. We bet you, too, will want to carry these principles of healthy eating forward for your long-term benefit.

Introducing Food Formulas

We admit it: we're big-time foodies. We looooooove food. And as practitioners, we go to the gut to treat almost everything. Food is just the best damn medicine. That's why we've made it the foundation of Yin Yang Reset. Not only is food cheaper and safer than Big Pharma, it's often faster and more effective.

Generations of TCM practitioners observed that each food has certain qualities that affect our bodies in specific ways. For example, they noticed that some foods heat the body, while others cool it. Some foods are drying, others hydrating. You might say that each food is programming your body to behave in a certain way.

Your body, too, has specific qualities. If you're experiencing fatigue, gut distress, or any other symptoms, this tells us that some of those qualities are out of balance. You may be deficient in one essential quality or have too much of another. Yin Yang Reset matches your body's imbalances with the foods known by TCM to bring them back into balance.

To help you determine your current constitution, we've got a handy little quiz (see page 20). Your quiz results will guide you to the Reset that's right for you and you'll be off and running. Each Reset is grounded in centuries of meticulous observation and analysis of how people respond to the foods they eat. We'll show you how to combine foods into specific "food formulas" to relieve your symptoms and rebuild your resilience.

Food formulas are the secret weapon in Yin Yang Reset. Every one of our recipes is built around one or more ingredients that have a track record for transforming specific symptoms. If you're familiar with herbal formulas, you'll know that each one has a main herb that drives the action to heal a symptom, along with supporting herbs that enhance that healing. That's how our food formulas work too.

As an example, let's look at our Garlic Chicken Drums recipe in the Blood-Building Reset. It's a phenomenal blood builder thanks to the three main healing foods: chicken, butter, and parsley. The chicken and parsley build blood, and both the chicken and butter are warming. While the other ingredients aren't on the Blood-Building food chart – that is, they aren't part of the formula – they won't interfere with the healing effects of the star ingredients. Their role is to create an irresistible flavour profile that helps you crave what heals you.

We invite you to ponder: What would it feel like to have all the energy you need to love your life, live your purpose, and help your family and community thrive? Read on and find out!

We're talkin' pep back in your step, baby. And we're thrilled to have you along for the ride.

Finding Your Reset with the QUIZ

Unlike Western medicine, Traditional Chinese Medicine (TCM) does not see you as a collection of separate organs and symptoms. TCM treats you as the dynamic interconnected system you really are. It aims for whole-body wellness, not just symptom relief.

As acupuncturists, we look beyond your symptoms to the root cause of what ails you. It's not about *what* you have, it's about *why*. That's why we ask our clinic patients a whole bunch of specific diagnostic questions about lifestyle, diet, emotions, and environment. We're super-nosy. Just knowing the name of a symptom or ailment is not enough.

For example, you may present to us with bloating, anxiety, or insomnia. But these are only WHAT is bothering you. Our question is, WHY? What else is going on in your life right now? Your insomnia is not the same as everyone else's. Likewise, each person's bloating or anxiety is unique.

TCM is the tool we use to help us navigate this landscape of "dis-ease" and search for nuances and patterns. Diseases do not exist in TCM, just imbalances. Once we find the root causes, we've got a map for your healing journey. Now we can get you back to feeling good again.

While we'd love to see each and every one of you in our clinic, we're even more stoked about giving you the tools to troubleshoot your own health issues. The very first tool we want you to use is our quiz.

The quiz is a cornerstone of the Yin Yang Reset. Think of it as your "practitioner on a page." It asks you many of the same nosy — um, diagnostic — questions we'd be asking if you came into the clinic. Doing the quiz will narrow down which Reset is right for you, right now.

If you're already seeing an acupuncturist or TCM practitioner, tracking is part of what they'll do for you. But if you're flying solo, you'll need a good "before" picture of your symptoms so you can see what's working.

Honestly, though, we encourage everyone to do the quiz, even if you *are* under the care of a practitioner. Not only does the quiz steer you to the right Reset, it allows you to stay in control and see how your symptoms and overall quality of life are shifting. Self-awareness through noticing and tracking your symptoms is one of the most powerful tools for change we know of. And it's free!

Tracking helps you make evidence-based choices, rather than just guessing your way along this journey to wellness.

So, before you start the Reset, do the quiz, either here in the book, or online.

We urge you to track your progress and be accountable for your health. Honour yourself for taking steps toward a better and healthier you. We know it's not easy, but the payoffs will be huge.

How to do the quiz

The quiz is organized into five sets of questions, one for each of the Resets:

- Blood Deficiency
- Dampness
- Qi Deficiency
- Qi Stagnation
- Yin Deficiency

To find your Reset, check YES for the symptoms you have experienced in the last 30 days. Even if you've had these symptoms in the past, report them ONLY if you've had them in this recent period.

Are you Blood Deficient?

1. Do you struggle to fall asleep? **YES NO**

2. Do you often feel fatigued? **YES NO**

3. Are you anemic or iron deficient? **YES NO**

4. Do you have a poor memory? **YES NO**

5. Are your nails, lips, and/or tongue pale in colour? **YES NO**

6. Do you have dry skin? **YES NO**

7. Do you have hair loss? **YES NO**

8. Do you sometimes have blurred vision or eye floaters? **YES NO**

9. Do you often feel dizzy or lightheaded? **YES NO**

10. Is your menstruation absent (amenorrhea) or less than 4 days long? **YES NO**

Do you have Dampness?

1. Do you have a lot of mucus or phlegm? **YES NO**

2. Do you have low energy or feel fatigued? **YES NO**

3. Do you experience bloating, lack of appetite, nausea and/or vomiting? **YES NO**

4. Are you carrying extra weight that's hard to lose? **YES NO**

5. Have you been told you are prediabetic or have insulin resistance? **YES NO**

6. Do you crave diet Coke/Pepsi/Soda? **YES NO**

7. Are your bowel movements frequently loose or alternating between loose and constipated? **YES NO**

8. Do you have symptoms of candida (yeast) or fungal infections? **YES NO**

9. Are you mentally foggy, overthinking and worrying a lot, or lacking motivation? **YES NO**

10. Do you have polycystic ovarian syndrome (PCOS)? **YES NO**

Do you have Qi Stagnation?

1. Do you feel "stuck" in life? **YES   NO**

2. Are you prone to feeling irritable, angry, unhappy, or frustrated? **YES   NO**

3. Do you get headaches or migraines or do you sigh frequently? **YES   NO**

4. Do you have dry, red, or irritated eyes? **YES   NO**

5. Do your symptoms get worse with stress or negative emotions? **YES   NO**

6. Do you feel like something is stuck in your throat, when there's nothing there? **YES   NO**

7. Do you have insomnia or have difficulty falling asleep and/or staying asleep? **YES   NO**

8. Do you grind your teeth, clench your jaw, or experience muscle or tendon pain, stiffness, or tightness, or rib cage soreness and tightness? **YES   NO**

9. Do you have body pain or discomfort that's worse on one side of your body? **YES   NO**

10. Do you experience any of the following: PMS (bloating, breast tenderness, and/or irritability), periods that stop and start, clotting, irregular menstrual cycles? **YES   NO**

Are you Qi Deficient?

1. Do you have low energy and feel fatigued or sluggish during the day? **YES   NO**
2. Have you been diagnosed with hypothyroidism? **YES   NO**
3. Do you find yourself overthinking, worrying a lot, or craving empathy from others? **YES   NO**
4. Do you feel exhausted in the afternoon, particularly after lunch? **YES   NO**
5. At the end of the day is your belly bloated (visibly distended)? **YES   NO**
6. Do you have food sensitivities and/or crave sweets? **YES   NO**
7. Do you experience burping, and/or gas and are your bowel movements frequently loose or alternating between loose and constipated? **YES   NO**
8. Do you bruise easily? **YES   NO**
9. Do you frequently catch colds and flus and recover slowly and/or do you sweat spontaneously, without exertion? **YES   NO**
10. Do you experience heavy periods and/or menstrual flow that is pale and/or watery? **YES   NO**

Are you Yin Deficient?

1. Do you feel tired and wired at the same time? — **YES   NO**
2. Do you get thirsty or have a dry mouth, with little desire to drink, or take small sips? — **YES   NO**
3. Do you startle easily and/or feel anxious or like your mind is racing? — **YES   NO**
4. Do you get red, flushed cheeks, especially in the afternoon or evening? — **YES   NO**
5. Do you have insomnia, with difficulty staying asleep? — **YES   NO**
6. Do you get night sweats? — **YES   NO**
7. Do you have a poor memory? — **YES   NO**
8. Do you have a hard time relaxing? — **YES   NO**
9. Are you frequently constipated? — **YES   NO**
10. Are you peri- or menopausal with hot flashes? — **YES   NO**

The quiz asks several questions about menstruation. If you're not menstruating, just skip these questions. Your results will not be skewed by not answering them.

Add up your quiz results from each section to see where you have the highest number of Yeses. The highest score is the Reset you should start with.

Many people get a nice, clear result and they're off and running. But what if two or more of your scores are so close you're not sure which Reset is the best? Don't worry, you'll just need to dig a little deeper. See "Help, my quiz results are not clear!" below, and we'll walk you through how to pinpoint your Reset.

After you've completed two weeks of the Reset (or longer), come back and redo the quiz to evaluate your changes.

Help, My Quiz Results Are Not Clear!

Let's say you've added up your scores and now you're confused because you have similar scores for one or more Resets. This is a common result. It just means you're going to have to do a little detective work to pinpoint the best Reset to start with.

We recommend reading the first few pages of each of the Resets for which you got similar scores. Here's where to find them:

- Blood Deficiency on page 53
- Dampness on page 105
- Qi Deficiency on page 163

- Qi Stagnation on page 223
- Yin Deficiency on page 283

Reading the intros to the relevant Resets can help you recognize where you're out of balance. As you're reading, notice which one really resonates. Which description names the symptoms that are bothering you the most? Ask yourself, if you could wave a magic wand, which symptoms would you most want to make disappear?

We've also included a case history for each Reset to give you a sense of what that particular imbalance can look like (for example, see page 54).

Take the quiz, do your reading, then go with your gut. Follow your chosen Reset for at least two weeks, maybe four, until you're noticing improvement. Then take the quiz again. If you still have lingering symptoms, see if your second-choice Reset will help correct them.

Remember, self-awareness and tracking are among the most powerful tools in your wellness toolbox.

Boost Your Reset with Movement, Hydration, Skin Brushing, and Sleep

Along with your food plan, we recommend some simple daily practices to support and speed your healing. Moving your body, proper hydration, skin brushing, and maximizing sleep are among our favourite tools for reaching optimal health.

Movement

Moving your body is essential for every Reset. Yes, food is medicine, AND so is movement. You'll find an activity guide tailored to your specific imbalance in each Reset.

Hydration

While we have no health advice for the *Walking Dead,* we'd like to point out that way too many of us are the *Walking Dehydrated*. Every molecular process in your body is affected by water. For example, when your water intake decreases, so does your cerebrospinal fluid. Your muscles get tired, your skin looks more dry and wrinkled, and you're more likely to be constipated.

But water is a funny thing. We've met people who full-on refuse to drink it unless it's been poured through ground coffee beans or processed into some kind of beverage – or, worse, an "energy drink" – that's really candy in disguise. People, please. Coffee is DEhydrating, and sugary drinks are … well, full of sugar, "flavourings," and other crap. That is NOT what we mean by hydration.

We're not saying it's easy to drink enough water. Tara once did a water challenge for a month. She documented it with pictures that showed how radiant her skin was by the end of the 30 days. She noticed that her nervous system was in check, and her digestion was flowing with ease. Yet, even after those tangible, documented results, she *still* finds it a struggle to drink enough water.

Sara is also doing her best to be an avid water drinker, but she has her own weird – let's call it "quirky" – approach: She frontloads her day with water. She'll consume two litres or more early in the day, often before 2 p.m., then sporadically drink throughout the evening.

Tara has a BIG thing about the kind of water she'll drink. If you serve her tap water, she'll take a pass. When we worked in the Village Community Acupuncture clinic together, in Vancouver, where the water is top notch, Tara refused to drink it, even after it had been boiled!

Unlike Tara, Sara will drink boiled water but she shares in Tara's refusal to drink tap water.

We both use Brita filters. We acknowledge that worrying about Vancouver's relatively pristine tap water is a First World Problem, but we figure why not avoid even small amounts of contaminants when it's this easy. Our water jugs sit on the counter, not in the fridge, because – get ready to hear this a million times – ice-cold drinks mess with the digestive system.

We're living in separate cities now, but we often call each other to troubleshoot the latest ache or pain. The first question we ask each other is "How much water have you had today?"

Which brings up the question: What *is* the magic number for how much water you should drink every day? Here's an easy equation for determining how much water YOUR body needs:

> **Your body weight in pounds ÷ 2 = your daily water consumption in ounces**
>
> For example, let's say you weigh 150 pounds:
>
> 150 ÷ 2 = 75
>
> *So, your ideal daily water consumption is 75 ounces.*
>
> Let's do it again, in metric this time:
>
> **Your body weight in kilos x 0.033 = your daily water consumption in litres**
>
> For example, let's say you weigh 70 kilograms
>
> 70 x 0.033 = 2.3
>
> *Your ideal daily water consumption is 2.3 litres.*

Hydration and your Reset

While everyone benefits from proper hydration, it is especially vital for the Blood and Yin Resets, because lack of hydration is at the root of those imbalances. Think of an engine that's constantly running at full speed, without rest or maintenance. It's going to get hot, dry up, and malfunction.

With Blood Deficiency, if you don't have the fluid to create the physical blood, even the right nourishment will not build you back up.

The same goes for Yin Deficiency: the less fluid in your body, the more you will dry out and heat up. You will feel like you're getting overheated and burning out at the same time. Hydration (as well as rest) will restore fluids to fuel you up and cool you down.

With Dampness, you probably resist drinking water because you already feel waterlogged. That's because the fluids are stuck and need to be mobilized and drained out. However, it's still important to drink fluids. Just make sure they're warm, as that will help to mobilize and drain the stuck fluids.

Skin brushing

Sara called Tara one day, when we were both going through a rough time. We diagnosed ourselves as both being in the Qi Stagnation category. This was based on the monumental amount of crap we were facing, including grief, sadness, loneliness, frustration, and burnout.

As per usual, we asked each other, "What are you doing each day to keep going?"

In unison, we piped up with, "I've been skin brushing." We agreed that it's an amazing way to keep our Qi moving. And in turn, moving Qi was helping us move through the tricky emotions life kept throwing at us.

Ancient cultures all over the world, from Egypt to the Americas, used some form of skin brushing to enhance their health. In China, for example, fruits and vegetables were dried into sponges much like the loofah sponges we use today.

Skin brushing is not just a fad. It's a practice that will keep your mind calm, your breasts a whole lot less tender, and your hormones on track. Stimulating your circulation and lymphatic system with this simple, gentle touch moves your Qi and keeps your healing on track. No stuck emotions in your body, and – double bonus! – your skin will take on a radiant glow.

Your skin is the largest organ in your body, and brushing is a great way to detox through that beautiful organ. Overall benefits include:

- Increasing circulation
- Improving digestion
- Creating glowing skin
- Enhancing lymph detoxification (which is also immune boosting)
- Reducing stress

Oh, and don't forget the all-important pleasure principle: skin brushing feels GREAT!

We're going to offer you two methods. First, there's the one you hear about most often, known as "dry skin brushing." Then, there's doing it in the shower. Yup, not dry at all. Let's call it wet brushing.

Guess which one we use? Rebels at heart, we brush our skin while we're in the shower. Because, honestly, if we have a free moment at night before bed, you can bet we are tucked in with a good book or our partner, NOT brushing our skin in the bathroom.

Wet brushing in the shower makes sense to us because:

- Multitasking, baby (yes, we know it's frowned upon, but life hacks are how we roll!)
- Saves dusting and vacuuming – who wants dead skin cells all over their bathroom? NOT US!
- Feels therapeutic to slough off the day and send all that gunk flowing down the drain
- Wet brushing first thing invigorates you and makes your clothes slide over your skin in the most glorious way. And who doesn't love to feel glorious?

We're always on the lookout for shortcuts. We want to make self-care so easy you can't say no to yourself.

How to do wet or dry skin brushing

Skin brushing is quick and easy, taking only a minute or two. First, choose your weapon. If you're dry brushing, use a natural bristle brush, loofah, or exfoliating mitt. If you're wet brushing, go for the mitt. That's what we use.

Follow this order:

1. Start at your feet and brush your skin upwards towards your heart using light circular motions.
2. Then start from your hands and go up your arms towards your heart. Focus on the areas that have a lot of lymph nodes: behind your knees, inner thighs, underarms, and neck (be gentle here)

Avoid brushing over varicose veins, your face, or any irritated skin.

Go ahead, grab a brush or mitt and get your glow on!

Sleep

Sleep as much as your body desires. For most people this falls between seven and nine hours. You will know you've had enough sleep when you wake up in the morning feeling rested and ready to roar. Can't remember that feeling? Read on to learn about the all-important sleep cycle.

You've probably heard the conventional wisdom that we should be in bed by 10 or 11 p.m. This makes sense from a whole lot of angles, but we find the TCM perspective particularly compelling.

If you're at all familiar with acupuncture, you've probably heard of meridians. There are 12 main meridians (channels or highways) that carry Qi, or energy, throughout your body. Each meridian feeds one of the 12 organ systems (which are associated with, but not limited to, our internal organs in Western medicine). Qi cycles through these meridians in a kind of circadian rhythm, every 24 hours.

Here's what can really up your sleep game: For quality sleep, the most important hours in this daily cycle are between 11 p.m. and 3 a.m. This is when Qi and blood are flowing most strongly through your gallbladder (11 p.m. to 1 a.m.) and liver (1 to 3 a.m.) organ meridians. Your liver is your body's main detoxifying organ. If you really want to maximize its ability to cleanse and rebuild your blood, you want to be asleep by 11 and well into a deep sleep by 1 a.m., the start of the two-hour liver cycle.

It's during these gallbladder/liver hours that your body basks in optimal rest and rejuvenation. So, if you're sitting up until 1:30 watching yet another Netflix episode, you're missing out on the most healing and restorative part of the sleep cycle.

When you first start sleeping more, you may want to sleep 10 to 12 hours a night. This is perfectly normal, so enjoy it! Being in an unbalanced state, you've likely been running on false energy (aka cortisol). As you begin to heal, stress hormones reduce and your body feels exhausted. Don't worry, you'll eventually catch up. As your stress hormones get replaced by actual energy, your body will regulate into a 7- to 9-hour sleep routine.

Why and How to Get Off Coffee

If a coffee detox — or even just the thought of it — hits you hard, that's a good sign you need to break up with coffee. Here's why we would like you to kick the coffee habit, at least during your Reset:

Stress — Traditional Chinese Medicine considers coffee overstimulating. This will increase your stress hormones, which will in turn add to the symptoms and angst you're already experiencing. Overstimulation means less REAL energy and a more restless mind and disturbed sleep.

Heat — In TCM terms, coffee produces heat in the body. Drinking too much (or even regular consumption, for some people) will heat up and dry out your body. If you're already overheated, coffee will make your symptoms even worse. This particularly affects Yin Deficiency and Qi Stagnation, the two Reset types that suffer from overheating.

Blood sugar and insulin — In Western terms, coffee can spike your blood sugar and insulin levels, especially if you're drinking it between, or instead of, meals. If you just can't let go of drinking coffee, then be sure to drink it with meals to avoid riding the blood-sugar roller-coaster all day, with every sip of coffee.

If you do feel ready to quit coffee, we applaud you! We know it's not easy, especially since you may feel worse before you feel better. Initially, you might experience mild headaches, brain fog, fatigue, irritability, and/or constipation. Fun times!

Coffee is a trickster. It can mask symptoms of fatigue and constipation. After your initial detox, you'll start to tune into your body and notice when you're tired or approaching burnout. Once you notice, you'll actually be able to DO something about it (for example, rest). This awareness will lead to deeper, more restful sleeps, a sustained level of calm energy, lower stress, and more balanced moods.

When you decide to quit, you'll have a spectrum of options. At one extreme is quitting cold turkey. If that's your style, go for it.

But we like gentler, more gradual approaches. Our top preference is to switch over to Dandy Blend, a caffeine-free herbal coffee substitute that is beneficial to your health and digestion.

If you're a die-hard coffee drinker, you might prefer scaling back by using decaf, for example:

Start by adding half decaf to your full-caf mug. Keep drinking the same amount of coffee, but slowly increase the amount of decaf until it's all you're drinking.

Then drink the same amount of all-decaf for two days.

The next step is to drink half the usual amount of coffee (now all decaf). If you still feel the need for a little kick, add some green tea. Then knock back to a quarter of your usual amount of coffee, or substitute with black or green tea.

Go ahead, give your body a boost by giving coffee the boot!

Foods to Avoid for All Resets

Genetically modified foods (GMOs)

Some people say genetically modified (GM) foods are safe to eat. We don't think so, and we recommend you avoid them.

Anecdotal evidence from human consumption has shown possible health issues including IBS, mood and sleep disorders, autoimmune diseases, diabetes, and autism.

Below is a list of ingredients that are derived from, and contain, GM foods. We believe it's essential to avoid these foods in their GM form. If you cannot find them as organic or non-GM, do not eat them. The effect of these GM foods is counterproductive to your health and can stall, if not reverse, all the good work you're doing.

- Alfalfa
- Corn
- Soybeans
- Canola oil
- Cottonseed oil
- Potatoes
- Papayas
- Sugar beets
- Zucchini (green and yellow)
- All animal products: eggs, milk, meat, gelatin

The Dirty Dozen

Why buy organic? Well, pesticides are toxic by design. They are created to kill living organisms such as insects, plants, and fungi. Some pesticides have been linked to a variety of health problems, including:

- Brain and nervous system toxicity
- Cancer
- Hormone disruption
- Skin, eye, and lung irritation

We recommend a handy little list called the "Dirty Dozen" from the Environmental Working Group (EWG). This list will help you avoid those fruits and vegetables with the highest levels of pesticide residues. We encourage you to purchase the organically grown alternatives when you can.

The EWG publishes an update of the worst offenders each year. It's worth checking the ewg.org website for changes. For example, in 2019 kale jumped onto the list for the first time, debuting in third place!

The EWG also provides the "Clean Fifteen," a list of fruits and veggies that are safer to buy non-organic because they have less pesticide residue. So, if money's an issue or you can't access organic where you live, reach first for the produce on the Clean Fifteen list.

You might ask, can't we just wash off the pesticides? Apparently not. Fruits you would normally wash, like apples and grapes, were washed before being tested, just as bananas were peeled. So, these ratings are based on the pesticide residue left on the produce after washing or peeling.

Here's the 2022 list of the Dirty Dozen. Buy organic if you can!

1. Strawberries
2. Spinach
3. Kale, collard and mustard greens
4. Nectarines
5. Apples
6. Grapes
7. Bell and hot peppers
8. Cherries
9. Peaches
10. Pears
11. Celery
12. Tomatoes

How Each Reset Rolls Out

You may be feeling like your energy has bottomed right out and you can't sink any lower. We've been there too. In fact, it's why we created Yin Yang Reset. We're inviting you to step on the Yin-Yang elevator and ride back up to the land of energy and clarity. Here's the plan.

Now that you've done the quiz, you know which Reset is right for you *at this time*. (Remember, this is a temporary reset to bring you back into balance, NOT a lifelong diet.) But before you begin, please read this section to get a feel for how each Reset rolls out. While the foods, recipes, and activities in each Reset are different, we have set them all up in the following way.

Each Reset kicks off with a quick dive into your particular imbalance – what it feels like, what causes it, and how you'll feel as the Reset brings you back into balance.

Then we walk you through the kinds of foods you'll be eating. The foods we recommend vary with each Reset, because each food has specific balancing powers. A food that strengthens one body may throw another body out of whack. This is the magic of Yin Yang Reset. Except it isn't magic, it's kitchen medicine.

Next, we give you a brief lowdown on exercise and other activities to rebalance your body, mind, and spirit. A few of our suggestions might even surprise you. Just like with food, some forms of exercise will build you up, while others drag you down.

Three Lists to Simplify Your Food Therapy

True confession: we love a list. A good list means you don't have to keep figuring out what to do, or in this case, what to eat. No more decision fatigue. We've got you covered with the following lists, unique to each Reset:

- **Food chart** – Your cheat sheet for choosing foods and beverages that have amazing healing powers to bring you back into balance.
- **Foods to avoid** – Don't worry, it's a short list!
- **Sample meal plans** – Four days of meal plans for each week (more about the meal plans coming up).

The Meal Plans and Recipes

We're pretty thrilled to be setting you up with a health FARMacy right in your own kitchen. But Yin Yang Reset wouldn't be worth a bean if the food was *just* for healing. Our wholehearted belief is that food should also be fun and enjoyable.

This is where the meal plans and recipes save the day. That fun factor can take a dive when you're faced with figuring out what to put on the table for dinner … and lunch … and don't forget breakfast. Three meals a day, seven days a week – plus, you'll be trying to use a bunch of ingredients that might be new to you. *Phew!*

A huge part of your success will be figuring out what a day of meals might actually look like. If this feels a teeny bit daunting, fear not. Get cozy with your food chart and recipes, and in no time at all you'll be intuitively wrangling your Reset's ingredients into deliciously healing food formulas.

Why have we mapped out only four days of meal plans for each week (plus a few extra dinners)? Well, in our experience, seven days of new recipes is just plain overwhelming, and we wouldn't do that to you. On the other days, make repetition your friend. Repeat your favourite recipes. You can also retrofit family recipes with ingredients on your food chart. Improvise and experiment, make the Reset fit you and your daily reality!

And that brings us to the heart and soul of your Reset: the yummy, healing recipes! Each Reset has its own rebalancing recipes for:

- 4 breakfasts
- 4 lunches
- 7 dinners
- 2 desserts

Without your familiar "go to's," you might sometimes feel like there's not much left to eat. We get that. But these recipes and meal plans will keep you groovin' all day long with yummy healing alternatives. Check your Reset's food chart for individual foods you can easily grab on the go, like an impromptu trail mix, or rice crackers and nut butter. Get curious and experiment. Expand your culinary horizons! Try weird stuff, you might like it.

Above all we want you to listen to your body. Some days you might need more protein. Other days you may be less hungry. Sometimes you just need some comfort food, and we've got recipes for that too. The best meal plans are built around food you love. Isn't it great to know that the foods in Yin Yang Reset will love you right back?

So, here's your Reset in a nutshell: Eat these foods and feel better. Plan, shop, cook, eat. Reheat the next day and eat again. Soon, you'll be reaching for the foods that are right for your body. You'll even get the hang of modifying your favourite recipes using Reset ingredients. Let your kitchen heal you.

Oh, and please break some rules. Instead of giving you a bunch of food rules to follow, we'd like to invite you to be a rule-breaker.

Why not have dinner for breakfast, leftovers for lunch, breakfast for dinner, and lunch for breakfast? Go ahead and double or triple that batch of handheld food and take it as a snack on the go.

POOF, you've got so many more options when you break the rules. Way to make life easier!

Give Yourself the Gift of a Bite-Sized Reset

We've done our best to make Yin Yang Reset easy for you. Now it's your turn to go easy on yourself. Sure, we want you to embrace all parts of the Reset because that's the best way to reboot your system. But, here's a little secret: half-assed is SO much better than nothing. Shrink down your Reset plan until you get this feeling in your bones:

Yup, I can do that!

Start with small goals that will give you solid success. If you're feeling overwhelmed by taking on the whole program, here are some tips for easing in (pick one or two that sound doable):

If this healing plan still sounds daunting, take a breath. You don't need to grasp the entire theory behind Yin Yang Reset for it to work. Just pick up a few foods from the food chart, choose a couple of recipes that make your mouth water, and dive in. Have fun shopping for new ingredients. Experiment and keep noticing how you feel.

That's it, you're doing it! And while we're on the subject of *easy does it,* who says you have to start a new program on a Monday? Go ahead, be a rebel. Start Yin Yang Reset on a Thursday evening or Saturday afternoon. Seize the moment and dive in. (But, always remember: half an ass is better than no ass at all!)

Yin Yang Reset Is Here When You Need It

We've emphasized that Yin Yang Reset is *short-term* food therapy. But even after you've completed two or more weeks on your Reset, it will still be there whenever you need it. Each Reset has the potential to support you whenever you need a boost.

For example, if you're feeling burned out or stressed, turn to the Qi Stagnation Reset to get things moving again. Add some condiments to your meals, like sauerkraut, brined pickles or lemons. Or grab a tall glass of kombucha for its rejuvenating sour property (and sparkly deliciousness).

If you're getting signals that your immune system is running on empty, turn to the Qi Deficiency Reset and sip some warming apple cinnamon teas, pull out your slow cooker for stews and casseroles, or roast up some root veggies or squashes.

Rinse and Repeat

We suggest you do the quiz again after two weeks on the Reset to track your progress. If your symptoms persist, continue for another two weeks. After four weeks, if you still have some residual symptoms, please reach out to us or visit your local acupuncturist. Some people stay on the plan for up to three months or longer.

Got questions? Check our FAQs and see if we've answered them. If not, get in touch. We're right here with you, ready to take you on this journey. Happy transformation, friend! You're here to heal and we are proud of you.

Are You Getting Enough Protein?

As you probably know, protein is one of the three macronutrients your body needs on the daily for optimal functioning. The other two macros are fats and carbohydrates; we'll go out on a limb and guess that you're getting enough of those. But what about protein? And what's with all the protein hype out there?

Protein provides your body with amino acids, which are the building blocks for muscle and other important structures, like the brain, nervous system, blood, skin, and hair. Protein also transports oxygen and other important nutrients throughout the body.

Let's see if we can clear a path through the confusion and help you figure out how much protein you should be eating.

First, we want to be clear that we're not here to debate plant-based versus animal proteins. We respect your choices. That's why we've worked hard to give you lots of choices in the recipes. Throughout each Reset you'll find a happy blend of vegetarian, vegan, and animal-based options.

We're also with all you vegans and vegetarians in both your ethical concerns and on the amazing healing power of plants. Like you, we enjoy beans and lentils, and make them part of our weekly rotation. Even so, we believe that reintroducing an animal-based protein can sometimes be beneficial for your health, especially if you're doing the Yin or Blood Reset.

So, whatever your choice of protein, we want to make sure you're getting enough of the stuff. Here's a quick calculation you can use to see how much protein *your* body needs each day.

Metric

> 0.8 X kilograms of body weight = grams of protein you need per day
>
> For example, if you are 85 kilos: 0.8 X 85 = 68 grams of protein.

Imperial

> 0.36 X pounds of body weight = grams of protein you need per day
>
> For example, if you are 150 pounds: 0.36 X 150 = 54 grams of protein.

Poof, you're a mathematician and a dietician all in one!

But what does 54 grams of protein look like? Here's a simple, tangible way to know you're getting enough: Make sure your plate has a hunk of protein on it – either plant-based or animal – as big as the palm of your hand. This way, you can be pretty sure you're getting the 20 to 30 grams of protein you need at each meal.

Our favourite protein powders

You'll notice that several of our recipes call for protein powder. They're an easy and digestible way to boost your intake. Flavour-wise, it's a bit of a game trying to find the one you like the most. Both of us keep two to four different kinds on hand for texture and flavour variety. Here are the ones we recommend.

All our recipes were tested with our top two choices, Genuine Health and Designs for Health, using their chocolate flavours. (Everything on our list is either vegan or vegetarian except for Designs for Health, which has beef protein. You can buy all these on Amazon.)

By far our favourite is Genuine Health Vegan Fermented Organic Proteins+ (Vanilla and Chocolate).

We also love Designs for Health PurePaleo Protein (beef protein) in the chocolate flavour. It tastes like hot chocolate!

Omega Nutrition Organic Pumpkin Seed Protein Powder is the cleanest choice, but not the best flavour.

- Genuine Health Vegan Fermented Organic Proteins+
- Designs for Health PurePaleo Protein
- Omega Nutrition Organic Pumpkin Seed Protein Powder

Hot Smoothies? Are You Kidding?

We are not kidding. In fact, we would like to claim the title "Hot Smoothie Queens."

If you've read this far, you'll know that cold foods can throw a wrench into your digestion, especially if your gut is already struggling. You need fire in your belly to break down and absorb the nutrients from your food, and cold foods put out that fire. That's why we are not fans of the ever-popular, so-called-healthy ice-cold smoothie.

But like everything else about Yin Yang Reset, this advice is not one size fits all. We are asking you to raise your own Smoothie Consciousness. If you have Qi Deficiency, hot smoothies are especially important. If it's cold outside, make 'em hot for sure. But in the summer months, you can try dialing your smoothies down to room temperature. Just be sure to watch for any bloating or feeling chilled inside, which means you should go back to the hot stuff and limit smoothies to two or three a week.

Here's how to master the art of the hot smoothie. First, combine the base ingredients. These will be the same for every smoothie, and every Reset. Now you're ready to supercharge the healing power of your smoothie by adding one or two ingredients from your Reset food chart. We've given you some examples below. Go ahead, experiment. You, too, can become a Hot Smoothie Queen. Or King, if you prefer.

Serves 1

Smoothie Base

- 1 cup almond milk
- 1–2 cups (depending on how thick you want it) HOT (just-boiled) water
- ½ green-tipped banana
- 2 tbsp ground flax
- 1 scoop protein powder (we like Genuine Health Vanilla flavour, but see page 48 for other options, or use your favourite)
- 1–2 scoops collagen (optional, for better results)

Reset additions:

- **Blood Deficiency:** Cherries, hemp seeds, organic kale, chard, spinach, red grapes, apricots
- **Dampness:** Pineapple, greens, ginger, flax oil, stevia, papaya
- **Qi Deficiency:** Strawberries, applesauce, ginger, cinnamon, dates
- **Qi Stagnation:** Citrus, green apple, strawberries and raspberries, microgreens, watercress, pumpkin and sunflower seeds
- **Yin Deficiency:** Raspberries, blackberries, blueberries, kiwis, hemp seeds

Part II
The Resets & Recipes

Blood Deficiency Reset

What's Happening in Your Body When Your Blood Is Deficient?

Your energy is low. Really low. You're not just "feeling a little tired." More like "drained by a vampire" or "down for the count." Welcome to Blood Deficiency! If you've ever had anemia, dizziness, blood loss (from injury, childbirth, or surgery), poor memory, pale complexion, or hair loss then you know what Blood Deficiency feels like.

From a Chinese-medicine perspective, your energy, or *Qi* (say *chee*), helps blood move through your body, nourishing your major organs and all the minor bits too. It's a symbiotic relationship: Qi and blood support each other. This is why your general sense of vitality, your get-up-and-go, takes a dive when your blood is deficient. You might look pale and have a dull complexion, experience dizziness, and suffer from insomnia. Life starts to feel like an uphill slog.

Deficient blood has mental and emotional consequences too. In Traditional Chinese Medicine, blood is seen as housing the mind, the home of consciousness. When blood is deficient, you'll notice your mind wanders and you feel ungrounded, forgetful, and exhausted. Emotionally, you might feel anxious or depressed.

Women are particularly vulnerable to Blood Deficiency. In fact, it underlies most female reproductive problems, from menstrual difficulties and infertility to postpartum exhaustion.

Among the many causes of Blood Deficiency are long-term illness, chronic stress, injury, surgery, and gastrointestinal bleeding. Unfortunately, deficiency can also be caused by worry and overwork. So maybe you don't want to work through the weekend or start a new business when your baby is two weeks old.

What deficient blood can look like

Tanner is in her twenties and is trying to conceive her first baby. She's been seeing a naturopath and is on supplements and receiving acupuncture. She and her partner have been checked out at a fertility clinic, and all signs (including sperm count) look good, but she is still not conceiving.

Here are the signs that Tanner needs to build her blood:

- Pale and tired
- Light, irregular periods

- Dry skin and hair, with some hair falling out
- Anxiety and chronic worrying
- Fuzzy thinking and memory problems
- Poor night vision and eye floaters

Working long night shifts has messed up Tanner's circadian rhythm. No wonder she's so tired.

What are the signs that the Blood-Building Reset is working for Tanner? While the best result would be to achieve pregnancy, building blood should also promote:

- Increased energy
- Sharper mind
- Greater sense of ease
- More colour in her complexion
- Periods more regular, with more normal flow
- Skin and hair more soft and supple, hair no longer falling out
- Better night vision

Goals for Building Blood

When your blood is deficient, you need to build it up. An abundance of blood brings you resilience and helps you feel the rhythmic pulse of life. Building your blood will lead to:

- Increased fertility
- More energy and mental focus
- Hormonal balance

In your current depleted state, you might feel like you're gazing up from the bottom of the energy abyss. But we promise, the Blood Building Reset, along with some key lifestyle practices, will transform you, body and mind. Prepare to be nourished from the inside out! As the fog of fatigue starts to lift, you might feel like you're waking up from a dream.

Let's explore how the Blood Building Reset works.

Kitchen Medicine for Building Blood

Here's the good news: The cure for Blood Deficiency is in the food you eat. Hippocrates had it right: "Let food be thy medicine and medicine be thy food."

We'll get you set up so everything you need to heal from Blood Deficiency is right there in your kitchen. We'll also encourage you to conserve and build energy through gentle exercise, meditation, yoga, and reconnecting with nature. But first, let's get you nourished.

The name of the game for the Blood Deficiency Reset is eating whole foods, specifically foods that are:

- Dark or red
- Sticky
- Hydrating

We want you to head to the dark side. Foods that are dark or red in colour are rich in chlorophyll and high in iron. *Think of it this way: foods that resemble the colour of blood, like beets, cherries, and red kidney beans, increase your blood production.* Dark green foods like chlorella, kale, and spinach contain chlorophyll, which ups the quantity and quality of red blood cells. Iron-rich foods like beef, molasses, and apricots are also excellent blood builders.

It might surprise you to know that, for building blood, how much and what you drink is as important as the foods you eat. If you don't have enough fluids to produce blood, you'll remain deficient no matter how much nutrition you add to your diet. (To find out how much water your body requires each day, check the hydration calculator on page 30.)

The temperature of what you eat and drink is important too. Think of your stomach as a cauldron where your digestive fire "cooks" your food and drink, breaking them down so you can absorb the nutrients. When you consume ice-cold foods and beverages, you're dousing that fire. This slows your digestion and leaves particles of food undigested, robbing you of nutrients your body needs to make new blood.

So, bid at least a temporary adieu to frozen treats like ice cream, cold drinks, and ice-cold smoothies. You'll also benefit from avoiding an excess of salad and other raw veggies. Raw food takes a lot more energy for your gut to break down. Even lightly cooking your veg will make it easier on your digestion, which will help you heal.

Bone broth, coconut water, and stout beer are powerful blood builders. Yes, that's right, you can enjoy up to three stout beers a week. Cheers! Be sure to let the beer sit on the counter for about 10 minutes first, to maintain that fire in your belly. Also, liver paté is like an iron supplement on a cracker. Our fave is chicken liver paté as a snack with small, round rice crackers.

As for grains, the most beneficial blood builders are oats, sticky rice, and mochi (a pounded sticky rice cake). The stickier the grain, the better, so make lots of rice pudding, risotto, oatmeal, and sticky rice veggie bowls. Thick, viscous, and high-protein foods like organic gelatin are blood-building powerhouses. That means real fruit juice gummies with gelatin are on the menu, yay!

Lastly, adding some minerals to your diet will help a lot. We love the ConcenTrace mineral drops added to daily water consumption. Also consider a good-quality whole iron supplement (if your blood work shows iron-deficient anemia), with added vitamin C, folic acid, and vitamin B12. Our favourite brand is Nature's Way Ultimate Iron softgels.

Eating foods like these will help get you building blood again so your mind and body can feel vibrant and clear.

Activities for Building Blood

When your blood is deficient, you are just tired. You want the energy to get moving, but if you manage to get outside and run for a week, that's it, you run right out of steam. We get it: everything seems hard because you get tired and winded so easily. But exercise is essential for your physical and emotional body. So, what can you do?

Here's the plan. Start slowly and work up to moving at least three times a week. But your key word for all activities is GENTLE. You build blood by slowing down, so avoid bootcamp for now.

Your best bet for building blood is low-intensity exercise that gets your blood moving. Aim for feeling energized but not exhausted. Here are some good options:

- Walking and hiking – extra points for getting out in nature and taking a friend
- Gentle yoga, like hatha, restorative, and yin
- Gentle swimming
- Cycling
- Slow dancing with a partner
- Slow sports like badminton, ping-pong, and 9-hole golf

Sun-bathing is also great for building blood, so grab that hat or sunscreen and get out there. Meditation is great too.

We have one last prescription for you that's an unparalleled blood-builder: hugs and cuddles. Put yourself in the path of love and fill up your love bucket every chance you get.

Beverages for Building Blood

Remember, your body can only build blood if you're well hydrated, so drink your medicine.

Daily green drink – One glass chlorella per day, following serving size on the bottle

Herbal coffee – Dandy Blend (we love this coffee substitute)

Coconut water – Buy 100 percent pure, not-from-concentrate. Our favourite brand is Taste Nirvana

Stout beer – Enjoy up to three a week (but not ice cold). Cheers!

Herbal and medicinal teas – See "How to make medicinal teas" on page 61. Traditional Medicinals have some great blood-building teas:

- Hawthorn with Hibiscus
- Nettle Leaf tea
- Burdock with Nettle Leaf tea
- Mother's Milk Shatavari Cardamom (amazing for all women, and men too)

How to Make Medicinal Teas

Making medicinal tea is almost as easy as boiling water. You won't be surprised to hear that step 1 is to boil some water.

The more tea bags you use and the longer you steep, the more medicinally potent your tea.

For most teas, use one tea bag for each cup (8 ounces) of water. If you're making just one cup, you can pop your tea bag right into the cup and pour the boiled water in. Or use your favourite teapot for larger quantities.

For steeping time, check the tea company's box to see what they recommend. Ideally, leave your tea to steep, covered, for at least 15 minutes. The longer, the stronger. Covering the infusion keeps any volatile oils in your tea, along with the tea's energetic warmth, for greater healing benefits.

If you want an extra-potent medicinal tea (especially helpful before bedtime), use 2 tea bags per cup of water and allow to steep for at least 20 minutes. (Beware, though, that longer steeping increases the chance your tea might taste a bit bitter, due to its medicinal phytochemicals.)

Blood Deficiency Reset Food Chart

Fruits	Vegetables	Grains
Apricots	Beets	Gluten-free oats
Blackberries	Broccoli	Mochi
Black currants	Cabbage	Quinoa
Blueberries	Carrots	Rice
Coconut flesh	Leafy greens	Spelt
Cooked fruits	Lettuce	Teff
Dates	Organic kale	
Figs	Organic potatoes	**Herbs**
Goji berries	Organic red peppers	
Lychee	Organic spinach	Nettles
Organic cherries	Organic Swiss chard	Parsley
Organic dark grapes	Sweet potatoes	
Raspberries		

Organic Protein	Additional	Foods to Avoid
Beef Black beans Chicken Eggs Kidney beans Lamb Liver Mussels Oysters Pinto beans Shrimp Tempeh Turkey	Black sesame seeds Hazelnuts Miso Nutritional yeast Organic butter Organic cow dairy Organic gelatin Organic goat dairy Organic molasses Organic peanuts Seaweed Sunflower seeds Virgin coconut oil Walnuts	Ice cold drinks/foods/smoothies Non-organic food GMO foods Alcohol* Too much raw food Coffee

* Stout beer is encouraged up to three times per week. Drinking cool is fine, but avoid drinking it ice cold straight out of the fridge.

Sample Blood-Building Meal Plans

Day 1

Breakfast: Cherry Almond Breakfast Bites & Cherry Kale Smoothie
Snack: Handful walnuts, dried figs, dried cherries, and cup of Hawthorn with Hibiscus tea
Lunch: Oven Baked Turkey & Avocado Wraps
Snack: Sesame rice crackers with liver pâté
Dinner: Glass Noodle Soup with Meatballs

Day 2

Breakfast: Leftover Glass Noodle Soup with Meatballs
Snack: Cherry Almond Breakfast Bites
Lunch: Beet Salad with Crumbled Goat Cheese & Mixed Greens
Snack: Organic Fruit Juice Gelatin Gummies
Dinner: Garlic Chicken Drums and leftover lunch Beet Salad

More Snack Options

- Thermos of miso soup with veggies and tofu and seaweed
- Orange Raspberry Muffins and glass of water with chlorella
- Baked organic kale chips and glass of coconut water
- Gluten-free toast with black sesame seed butter, honey, and cinnamon
- Ginger Molasses Cookies and cup of Mother's Milk Shatavari Cardamom Tea

Day 3

Breakfast: Cherry Kale Smoothie
Snack: Gluten-free toast with sunflower seed butter topped with raisins and cinnamon
Lunch: Kale Chickpea Raisin Salad
Snack: Mixed berries and organic grapes and a cup of Nettle Leaf tea
Dinner: Mango & Black Beans in Coconut Lime Sauce

Day 4

Breakfast: Orange Raspberry Muffins & Cherry Kale Smoothie
Snack: Organic peanut butter and rice crackers and a cup of Nettle Leaf tea
Lunch: Smoked Fakin' Bacon Club Sandwich
Snack: Couple pieces mochi and a cup of Hawthorn with Hibiscus tea
Dinner: Mixed Bean & Beef Chili

More Snack Options

- Cherry Almond Breakfast Bites and glass of room temperature water with Trace Mineral Drops
- Trail mix with walnuts, hazelnuts, sunflower seeds, dried goji berries, apricots, and raisins
- Thermos of bone broth

Blood-Building Breakfasts

Cherry Almond Breakfast Bites

These little goodies are as easy to make as they are nourishing. Make them small or cookie size – and, yes, go ahead and smile 'cause you're eating a cookie for breakfast! They're a perfect snack to take on the go and pop in your mouth when you're feeling hangry. Double up on the cherry power and pair these with the Cherry Kale Smoothie on page 73 to hit your daily protein quotient.

Substitution tip: You can replace the almond butter with organic peanut butter.

Makes 1 dozen

- » 2 very ripe bananas, mashed (riper = better flavour)
- » 2 tbsp almond butter
- » 1 tbsp raw honey
- » 1 cup quick-cooking rolled oats
- » ½ cup dried organic cherries (or raisins, chopped dried apricots, or dried raspberries or blackberries)

1. Preheat the oven to 350°F and grease a baking sheet with butter or coconut oil, or cover in parchment paper.
2. In a medium bowl, mash the bananas with a fork or potato masher until almost smooth (some lumps are okay). Stir in the almond butter and honey until well combined.

3. Add the rolled oats, mixing well, then toss in the dried cherries or other dried fruit. Stir until combined.
4. Spoon the mixture onto the baking sheet in your preferred size and bake for 15 to 20 minutes, or until lightly browned. Allow to cool on the baking sheet before enjoying with a hot cup of tea.

Hazelnut Goji Yogurt with Drizzled Honey

When you're running on fumes, the very thought of making breakfast can feel daunting. That's why we love this recipe. Toss it in a bowl and, voila, it's ready — fast and easy, like a healthy bowl of cereal. The goji berries are the pièce de résistance, with their ruby-red colour and candy-like chew.

Ingredient tip: Add variety by tossing in oat granola clusters.

Protein tip: To bump up your breakfast protein, sprinkle in 1 to 1 1/2 tablespoons of pumpkin seed protein powder (defatted ground pumpkin seeds).

Serves 1

- 1 cup organic plain yogurt (goat or cow milk)
- ½ banana, sliced
- ¼ cup roughly chopped hazelnuts
- 2 tbsp dried coconut flakes
- 1 tbsp goji berries
- drizzle of raw honey
- sprinkle ground cinnamon

1. Place your yogurt in a bowl and top with the banana slices, hazelnuts, goji berries, and a drizzle of delicious honey sprinkled with cinnamon.

Orange Raspberry Muffins

Dear teff, we love you. Please stay in our rotation forever. Like all our muffins, these are easy to make and full of nourishment. We jokingly call these "Magic Muffins" because when people taste them, they can't believe these little treats are part of a healing diet. So, get out there and spread the word … er, the muffins!

Protein Tip: To meet your protein needs, pair with our Cherry Kale Smoothie on page 73.

Teff tip: Tiny whole-grain teff has been a staple of the Ethiopian diet for thousands of years. It is high in iron, protein, and vitamin C, the perfect combination for replenishing blood. Teff can be used in baked goods like pancakes and muffins and also makes a great hot cereal.

Makes 1 dozen muffins

- 1½ cups teff flour (we use Bob's Red Mill)
- ½ cup tapioca flour
- 2 tsp baking powder
- ½ tsp baking soda
- 2 tbsp chia seeds, ground in a coffee grinder or Vitamix
- 2 organic eggs
- 2 bananas, mashed
- 1 cup almond (or coconut) milk
- ⅓ cup melted organic butter
- ½ cup coconut palm (or organic) sugar
- zest of one orange
- 1 cup raspberries (fresh or frozen)

1. Preheat the oven to 350°F and grease a 12-cup muffin tin, or do as we do and line with paper cups.
2. In a medium bowl, combine the flours, baking powder and soda, and the ground chia.
3. In a large bowl, beat the eggs. Combine with the bananas, milk, melted butter, sugar, and orange zest.
4. Slowly add the dry ingredients into the wet and stir until combined. Fold in the raspberries.
5. Pour batter into the prepared muffin tin and bake for 30 minutes, or until a knife inserted in the middle comes out clean. Cool on a wire rack and enjoy.

Cherry Kale Smoothie

YES, we know you want to jump into your Reset with both feet, but easy on the kale to start! Also, remember that ice-cold drinks can weaken your digestive "fire." You need your gut to be functioning optimally to break down your food and produce blood. Your best bet is to drink this smoothie at room temperature. (Get the full story on smoothies on page 49.)

Kale tip: Start with ¼ cup of kale and increase as your palate becomes accustomed to the strong flavour of this lively, nourishing food.

Protein tip: For the protein powder, we like the taste of Genuine Health Vanilla, but use your favourite (see page 48 for our lowdown on protein powders).

Serves 1

- ½ banana, cut into chunks
- ½ cup organic cherries, pitted
- ½ cup organic kale, thick ribs removed, leaves torn into pieces
- 1 cup almond (or coconut) milk
- 1-2 cups room temperature water (depending on how thick you like it)
- 1 scoop protein powder

1. In your blender or Vitamix, combine ingredients and blend until smooth (about 30 seconds). If it's ice cold, allow it to warm up to room temperature before drinking.

Blood-Building Lunches

Oven-Baked Turkey & Avocado Wraps

You build blood by slowing down. Getting wrapped up in the nonsense of daily living depletes your blood. But wrapping up your food in a delicious tortilla? That's the way to build blood! In less than 5 minutes, "it's a wrap," leaving you plenty of time to chill out and enjoy.

Wrap tip: Try a variety of gluten-free wraps and find your favourite. We love coconut, cassava, and dehydrated veggie wraps. Find them at your local health food store (check the frozen food section).

Serves 2

- » 2 brown rice tortilla wraps (we use Food For Life brand)
- » 6 slices organic oven-baked turkey
- » organic baby spinach
- » 1 organic tomato, diced
- » 1 avocado, sliced
- » Dijon mustard

1. Preheat the oven to 350°F.
2. Heat the tortilla wraps in the oven for a minute or two, until warm but still soft.
3. Spread a little mustard on each wrap and top with 3 slices of turkey, a handful of baby spinach, diced tomato, and avocado slices.
4. Wrap up and enjoy a quick-and-easy lunch.

Beet Salad with Crumbled Goat Cheese & Mixed Greens

Cultivating blood-building kitchen practices will have you feeling vibrant again. And since nothing feeds blood better than the majestic beet, we recommend cooking up a large batch at the beginning of the week. That way, you can toss together a meal like this in 10 minutes, flat! While you're at it, double or triple the dressing by shaking it up in a large jar to enjoy this all week long.

Protein tip: Add leftover chicken/salmon/hard-boiled eggs from the night before as a side.

Serves 2

Beets
- » 3 medium–large beets, boiled
- » ½ tsp salt

Dressing
- » 4 tbsp olive oil
- » 2 tbsp balsamic vinegar
- » 1 tbsp grainy Dijon mustard
- » salt and freshly ground black pepper, to taste

Salad
- » 4 cups mixed greens
- » ½ small red onion, very thinly sliced
- » 4 tbsp soft organic goat cheese

1. Scrub the beets and put them in a large saucepan with the ½ tsp salt and water to cover by 2 inches. Bring to a boil and cook for about 45 minutes, until

tender when pierced with a fork. Drain and cool. Once cool enough to handle, peel off the skins with a paper towel.
2. For the dressing, combine all the ingredients in a jar. Put the lid on and shake until well blended.
3. To serve, cut the beets into bite-sized chunks. Divide the salad greens onto two plates and arrange the beets on the greens. Top with the onion slices and crumbled goat cheese. Drizzle 1 tablespoon of dressing over each salad and season with salt and pepper.

Smoked Fakin' Bacon Club Sandwich

"Wow, it actually tastes like bacon. I would eat this again," says everyone at your table. Tempeh is a savoury fermented soy product that also happens to be an excellent blood builder. Pair it with a handful of chlorophyll-rich spinach to bring out your inner Popeye. Toot toot!

Serves 3

- » 1 package organic smoked tempeh (look for smoked or bacon flavour)
- » 1 tsp olive oil
- » 6 slices brown rice (or other gluten-free) bread
- » honey mustard (or Dijon or grainy mustard with a bit of raw honey added)
- » 1 organic tomato, sliced
- » 1 avocado, sliced lengthwise
- » few handfuls organic baby spinach
- » sea salt and freshly ground black pepper, to taste

1. Slice the tempeh very thin (about ⅛ inch). In a medium frying pan, heat the oil over medium heat and fry the tempeh slices for about 1 to 3 minutes on each side, until golden brown.
2. Toast the bread slices, spread with the mustard, and top with the tomato, avocado, spinach, and cooked tempeh slices.

Kale Chickpea Raisin Salad

We wanted to call this Deconstructed Blood-Building Formula, but we worried it might not sound as tasty. Just so you know, though, this recipe has all the components of the ultimate blood-building dish. Chlorophyll-rich ingredient? That would be the kale. Vitamin C? Yup, the orange pepper. Iron? Got the raisins. But, wait, what about protein? Oh, right, that's covered by the chickpeas. Voilà, you've got a food formula that tastes great and heals what ails you.

Digestion tip: Whip this up the day before to allow the dressing to tenderize the kale. The acid almost "cooks" the raw kale, making it WAY easier to digest. This means you can better absorb the nutrients you need so you can get better faster.

Serves 4

- » 4 cups organic kale, chopped into bite-sized pieces
- » 2 tbsp olive oil
- » 14-oz can organic chickpeas
- » 1 small organic orange pepper, diced into ½-inch pieces
- » ½ cup organic raisins
- » 1½ tbsp apple cider vinegar
- » 1 clove garlic, minced
- » sea salt and freshly ground black pepper, to taste

1. Wash and dry the kale pieces and put them into a large salad bowl. Drizzle with 1 tablespoon of the olive oil and massage with your hands until the leaves soften and turn a rich emerald green.
2. Toss in the chickpeas, pepper dice, and raisins and mix together.
3. Drizzle on the remaining 1 tablespoon of olive oil and the vinegar. Add the garlic, salt, and pepper, and toss until well combined.

Avocado & Goat Cheese Burrito

The three heavy hitters in this dish are kale, eggs, and goat cheese, nutrient-dense foods that quickly replenish your blood. Whip up this easy recipe to slow down a busy day with a quiet sit-down lunch.

Wrap tip: Try a variety of gluten-free wraps and find your favourite. Along with corn and rice, we love coconut, cassava, almond flour and dehydrated veggie wraps. Find them at your local health food store (check the frozen foods).

Serves 4

- 1-2 tbsp olive oil
- 1 small onion, diced
- 1 cup sliced mushrooms
- 3 cups finely chopped organic kale
- 5 organic eggs
- pinch sea salt and freshly ground black pepper
- 4 gluten-free corn or rice tortillas

Toppings
- organic cherry tomatoes
- avocado slices
- organic salsa
- goat cheese

1. Preheat the oven to 350°F.
2. In a large frying pan, heat the olive oil over medium heat and sauté the onion for 2 minutes. Add the mushrooms and cook for 3 to 5 minutes, until the vegetables are tender. Stir in the kale and cook for a couple of minutes, until the leaves are soft and wilted.
3. In a medium bowl, beat the eggs. Pour them into the pan and sprinkle with salt and pepper. Cook, stirring gently, until the eggs are fluffy and done as you like.
4. To serve, heat the tortillas in the oven for a minute, until warm but still soft. Spoon the egg mixture onto each tortilla, add your favourite toppings, roll up, and enjoy!

Blood-Building Dinners

Mango & Black Beans in Coconut Lime Sauce

This recipe is our hats-off to a little Vancouver restaurant that dared to be different. The dish stayed with us long after the restaurant shut its doors, and now we've modified it for maximum blood-building properties. The delicious combo of hearty black beans and sweet mango with a twist of lime makes this a weekday staple, especially since it can be whipped up in less than 30 minutes.

Serves 4

- » 1 can full-fat organic coconut milk (we like Native Forest)
- » 2 tbsp raw honey
- » 2 cups frozen mango chunks
- » zest and juice from ½ lime
- » 14-oz can organic black beans
- » ¼ tsp salt
- » cooked jasmine rice, for serving

1. In a large frying pan over medium-high heat, whisk together the coconut milk, honey, and salt and bring to a low boil. Reduce the heat and simmer, stirring occasionally, for 5 to 10 minutes.
2. Add the mango and lime zest and continue to simmer and stir for about 10 to 15 minutes, until the volume is reduced by half.
3. Stir in the lime juice and beans, and cook for another 5 minutes.
4. Serve over rice.

Ruby Red Beet & Beef Borscht

If there's one recipe you make over and over again, let it be this blood-building powerhouse. Blood is created deep within the bones, beets are grown deep in the soil. Align your inner vitality with the pulse of the earth.

Serves 4-5

- » 2 tbsp olive oil
- » 1 lb organic stewing beef, chopped into 1-inch cubes
- » 1 large onion, chopped
- » 3 carrots, roughly chopped
- » 1 clove garlic, minced
- » 3 tbsp apple cider vinegar
- » 8 cups organic beef broth
- » 3 large beets, peeled and chopped into ½-inch cubes
- » 4 cups thinly sliced red cabbage
- » 1 large organic Yukon gold potato, chopped into ½-inch cubes
- » ½ cup minced fresh dill (plus more for garnish)
- » sea salt and freshly ground black pepper, to taste
- » optional: organic sour cream

1. In a large pot over medium heat, warm one tablespoon of the oil and brown the beef cubes (about 5 minutes). Transfer to a plate and set aside.
2. Add the remaining tablespoon of oil to the pot and sauté the onion and carrots over medium heat for 3 to 5 minutes. Stir in the garlic and cook for another minute.
3. Pour in 2 tablespoons of the apple cider vinegar to deglaze the pot. Return the browned beef to the pot along with the beef broth and beets. Bring to a boil, reduce to a lively simmer and cook, covered, for 1½ to 2 hours, until the beef is tender.
4. Stir in the cabbage, potato, and dill and simmer, covered, for an additional 30 minutes.
5. Season to taste with the last tablespoon of apple cider vinegar, salt, and pepper (though if your beef broth is salted, you might not need to add salt).
6. Spoon into bowls, top with a dollop of sour cream if you like, and sprinkle with the dill.

Fragrant Red Curry Mussels

Learning to cook with new ingredients can be a challenge, but this one is fun. Having friends over? Double the recipe, place it in the middle of the table, and break (gluten-free) bread together. They'll never know you're on a "diet"!

Beverage tip: This is a great meal to serve with a tall glass of stout beer.

Serves 3

- » 2 lb fresh mussels
- » 3 tbsp organic butter
- » 2 cloves garlic, minced
- » 1 tbsp minced or finely grated ginger root
- » 1 can organic coconut milk
- » 3 tbsp red curry paste
- » ½ cup minced cilantro
- » juice and zest of 2 organic limes (top layer only, not the bitter white part underneath)
- » gluten-free or spelt bread, for serving

1. To prepare the mussels, put them in a large colander in the sink. If they have beards, pull them out. Discard any shells that have cracks along with any open shells that don't close up when you tap them on the counter. Wash each mussel in cold water to remove any debris.
2. In a large pot, melt the butter over medium heat. Add the garlic and ginger and sauté for 1 minute, stirring frequently.

3. Raise the heat to high and whisk in the coconut milk and curry paste. Bring to a simmer and add the mussels. Cover the pot, reduce the heat to medium-high, and cook, stirring occasionally, for 5 to 8 minutes or until the mussels open.
4. Remove from the heat and stir in the cilantro and the lime zest and juice.
5. Serve into individual bowls and enjoy.

Sweet Potato Fritters with Smashed Avocado

YESSSS, fritters for dinner! Instead of frying these little puppies, you retain the blood-nourishing power of the sweet potato, eggs, carrots, and cheese by baking them. Serve alongside a spinach salad for a tasty dinner, or take on the go as a snack or lunch.

Batch tip: Seriously, these are so fast, easy, and yummy, you might want to double-batch 'em.

Makes 12-16 fritters

Fritters
- » 2 large sweet potatoes, grated (about 4 cups)
- » 2-3 large carrots, grated (about 2 cups)
- » 4 organic eggs
- » ½ cup grated organic goat cheddar
- » 2 scallions, chopped
- » 1 tsp oregano
- » 1 tsp cumin
- » 1 tsp salt
- » freshly ground black pepper
- » ¼ cup tapioca flour

Smashed Avocado
- » 1 avocado
- » juice of 1 lime
- » 1 tsp olive oil
- » salt and freshly ground black pepper, to taste

1. Preheat the oven to 425°F and line a baking sheet with parchment paper.
2. Pile the grated sweet potato and carrots onto a clean dish towel. Roll them up and wring out as much liquid as possible over the sink. The more you squeeze out, the crispier the fritters will be.
3. In a large bowl, beat the eggs. Stir in the cheddar, scallions, oregano, cumin, salt, and pepper. Add the grated sweet potato and carrots. Sprinkle on the tapioca flour and combine well.
4. Scoop the mixture onto the prepared baking sheet in 12 to 16 small rounds and flatten with the back of a spoon. You'll probably need to spread them over 2 baking sheets or bake in 2 batches. Bake for 30 minutes, until the fritters look set.
5. Meanwhile, mash the avocado in a small bowl and combine with the lime juice and olive oil. Season with salt and pepper.
6. Serve the fritters topped with a scoop of the smashed avocado.

Glass Noodle Soup with Meatballs

Soups are excellent blood-builders, giving you that extra pep in your step. Glass noodles are fun to slurp, meatballs add a delightful texture, and carrots and kale add a little zest. Slurp up and smile! We're pretty sure this'll become a mainstay in your dinner rotation.

Noodle tip: Longkou Vermicelli is a common brand of mung bean noodles found in the international section of most grocery stores. If you can't find it, rice noodles will substitute nicely.

Serves 4

Meatballs
- 1 lb ground organic chicken or turkey
- 1 organic egg, beaten (optional)
- 1 garlic clove, minced
- ¼ cup minced cilantro
- ½ tsp sea salt
- freshly ground black pepper
- 3-5 tbsp brown rice (or any gluten-free flour)
- 2 tbsp olive oil

Soup
- 8 cups organic chicken broth
- 2 carrots, thinly sliced
- 3 cups finely chopped organic kale
- 3 bunches mung bean vermicelli (cellophane noodles)

1. In a medium bowl, combine the ground meat, egg, garlic, cilantro, salt, pepper, and flour. Roll into about 16 1-inch meatballs.
2. In a large frying pan, heat the olive oil over medium heat and brown the meatballs on all sides. Remove from the pan and drain on a paper-towel-lined plate.
3. In a large pot, bring the broth to a boil. Add the browned meatballs, reduce the heat, and simmer for 10 minutes.
4. Add the carrots and vermicelli and cook for another 4 minutes. Stir in the kale and turn off the heat. Serve immediately!

Mixed Bean & Beef Chili

Who doesn't love a piping hot bowl of chili? We sure do! And since chili always tastes better the next day, why not whip this up on Sunday night for a quick-and-easy weeknight meal you can heat up in a flash. The classic combo of beans, beef, and molasses makes for a highly therapeutic and super-tasty dish.

Serves 4

- 3 tbsp olive oil
- 1 lb organic extra-lean ground beef
- 1 large onion, chopped
- 1 organic yellow bell pepper, chopped
- 3 cloves garlic, minced
- 3 14-oz cans organic diced tomatoes, with liquid
- 1 14-oz can organic mixed beans, drained and rinsed
- 1 14-oz can organic black beans, drained and rinsed
- ½ tsp organic molasses
- 1 tsp dried oregano
- 1 tsp ground cumin
- ¼ tsp ground coriander
- ¼ tsp ancho chili powder
- ⅛ tsp chipotle chili powder
- 1 tsp sea salt
- freshly ground black pepper

1. In a large pot, heat one tablespoon of the oil over medium heat. Add the ground beef and brown, stirring frequently (about 5 minutes). Remove from the pan and set aside.
2. In the same pan, heat the remaining oil over medium heat and sauté the onion and bell pepper until the onion is translucent (about 5 minutes). Add the garlic and cook for an additional minute.
3. Return the browned beef to the pot along with the tomatoes with their liquid, and the beans, molasses, and spices, including a generous grind of black pepper. Bring to a boil, reduce to a simmer, and cook, covered, for 1 to 1½ hours, stirring occasionally.
4. Serve, slurp, and savour!

Garlic Chicken Drums

OMG, we love this dish. There's something heartwarming about the sizzling combo of butter and garlic. The aroma alone attracts a gathering, so consider doubling or tripling the recipe. Plus, once you've tasted it, you'll want extra for leftovers and lunches. The fresh herbs and organic chicken drumsticks are key to building your blood. Serve with oven-baked sweet potatoes and a light, mixed green salad drizzled with olive oil and balsamic vinegar.

Serves 3

- » 6 organic chicken drumsticks
- » sea salt and freshly ground black pepper, to taste
- » 1 tbsp olive oil
- » 1 tsp organic butter
- » 1 tbsp rice (or apple cider) vinegar
- » 2 cloves garlic, minced
- » ½ cup minced parsley

1. Preheat the oven to 375°F.
2. Season the drumsticks with a sprinkling of salt and pepper.
3. In a large oven-proof frying pan, heat the olive oil and butter over medium-high heat and brown the drumsticks on all sides, about 5 to 6 minutes.
4. Cover the frying pan with a lid (or tinfoil) and bake for 30 minutes, or until the chicken is cooked.

5. Remove from the oven and pour in the vinegar, minced garlic, and parsley. Toss to coat and let sit for a few minutes to marry the flavours. And believe us when we say, it's a VERY happy marriage.

Blood-Building Desserts

Ginger Molasses Cookies

Hello, sweet tooth, where have you been? These little gems build blood and make you want to hug the person next to you. The secret blood-building ingredients? Iron-rich teff and molasses.

Baking tip: Molasses has a tendency to burn, so keep an eye on these while they're baking to avoid burning their bottoms.

Makes 2 dozen cookies

Dry
- 1½ cups teff flour (we use Bob's Red Mill)
- ½ cup tapioca flour
- 2 tsp ground ginger
- 2 tsp ground cinnamon
- ½ tsp ground cloves
- 1 tsp baking soda

Wet
- 2 tbsp chia seeds, ground in a coffee grinder or Vitamix
- ⅓ cup hot water
- ½ cup organic butter, room temperature
- ½ cup coconut palm sugar (or organic sugar)
- ⅓ cup organic molasses

1. Preheat the oven to 350°F and line a baking sheet with parchment paper.
2. In a medium bowl, combine the dry ingredients.

3. In a small bowl or measuring cup, whisk together the chia seeds and hot water and let sit for a minute.
4. In a large bowl, cream together the butter and sugar with an electric mixer. Beat in the molasses and sticky chia mixture until well combined.
5. Slowly add the dry mixture into the wet, stirring well until a thick dough is formed.
6. Drop the dough onto the prepared baking sheet by the spoonful (or roll into 1-inch balls) and flatten slightly. Bake for 7 to 14 minutes. Let cool on a rack before hollering "It's cookie time!"

Ginger Oat-Crusted Baked Pears

This warm and inviting spin on apple crisp begs to be showcased all year long, not only during the winter months. It will fill your belly with all the therapeutic properties of oats, that magnificent blood restorer. Enjoy this as a treat after dinner, or even for a weekend brunch. Trust us, your body will thank you!

Coconut cream tip: Refrigerate the can of coconut milk for a couple of hours or overnight, so the cream separates from the water. Carefully open the can and scoop out the thick, delicious cream on top.

Serves 4

- » 2 firm, ripe organic pears (like Bosc)

Oat crust
- » ½ cup old-fashioned rolled oats
- » 2 tbsp coconut palm (or organic brown) sugar
- » 2 tbsp organic butter (or virgin coconut oil)
- » 1 tbsp shredded coconut
- » 1 tsp finely grated ginger root
- » 1 tsp ground cinnamon
- » ½ cup water
- » organic vanilla yogurt or coconut cream (full-fat coconut milk), optional for topping

1. Preheat the oven to 375°F.
2. Slice the pears lengthwise. Use a spoon to scoop out the seeds and core. Place core-side up in an 8 by 8-inch baking dish.
3. In a small bowl, crumble together the crust ingredients with your hands to evenly distribute the butter or oil.
4. Mound the oat mixture into the pear halves.
5. Pour the ½ cup of water into the bottom of the baking dish and bake for about 40 to 50 minutes, until the pears are crisp-tender when pierced with a knife.
6. Delicious on their own or topped with a dollop of organic vanilla yogurt or coconut cream.

Dampness Reset

What's Happening in Your Body with Dampness?

Do you feel like you're trudging through the mud, with a big "out of order" sign on your back? We get it. You've landed yourself in one of the trickiest health patterns in Traditional Chinese Medicine, known as Dampness.

TCM describes Dampness as an accumulation of sludge and toxins. That may sound straightforward, but it's not. Damp is a combo platter of a few health patterns involving all your major organ systems. It's hard to even know where to start because Damp is a mashup of many imbalances – Qi Deficiency and Stagnation – with Damp piled on top.

With Dampness, everything is heavy and stuck and wants to stay that way. If you've noticed an inner resistance to movement and change, that's Damp being the boss of you.

Physically, Damp can show up as a heavy, tired, sluggish feeling. You may have a noticeable lack of appetite, carry extra weight you can't seem to lose, or have candida or edema. Even a glass of water might make you feel bloated. You might get colds that trail off into lingering sinus congestion and excess mucus.

Mentally, you may struggle with a foggy brain that robs you of clarity and focus. Emotionally, you might experience negative self talk, lack of motivation, depression, anxiety, and/or feeling apathetic about taking care of yourself.

Which leads us to the Big Question: WTF? How and when did this Damp pattern show up and, while we're at it, why? Let's look to your history for clues.

As a child, did you take round after round of antibiotics for repeated ear infections? Was your family home unstable, depriving you of the support, love, and nurturing you needed? What about those turbulent teen and young adult years: who was there to guide and truly listen to you and how did you soothe yourself? And, more recently, are you "supermom," sacrificing your own needs and health for your family?

The cause of Dampness is more likely a cascade of events over time than any single experience, but whatever got it started, we'd like you to know that IT'S NOT YOUR FAULT.

Maybe you've said to yourself, if only I wasn't so lazy, if only I could control what I eat, if I could just exercise more, and really get it together for once ...

But we don't buy the shame game. For one thing, as you've probably noticed, shame is NOT a healing force. Also, your current state of Dampness is a logical response to REAL events in your life, and you have been coping to the best of your abilities.

You heard us: you're doing everything right, so you can let go of all that shame and guilt. Somewhere along the line your gut-brain connection got severed. This means that, in spite of your best efforts, the food you eat gets shoved away in the "closet" (aka fat cells) instead of being used as fuel to energize you. This is why all the fad diets that seem to work for everyone else do NOT work for you.

When you have Dampness, you're starving in the midst of plenty. The cause is unique to each person, but the bottom line is that your gut and brain are not on speaking terms and your digestion no longer functions optimally.

What dampness can look like

Trish is in her mid-forties, and she has issues. Lots of issues. She works hard at taking care of herself. She eats organic and cooks at home, and is usually following the latest diet. She's been to see boatloads of specialists and alternative practitioners. But nothing seems to work.

Here are the signs that Trish needs the Dampness Reset:

- Low energy
- Hormonal issues, like estrogen dominance, irregular heavy periods, and PCOS
- Sluggish digestion – constipation, stinky gas, burping, bloating, suspected candida
- Weight struggles
- Skin rashes
- Low thyroid
- Foggy brain
- Edema in feet and general puffiness

Trish is frustrated that she eats the same amount of food as her slimmer friends and ends up 40 pounds heavier. Not to mention working this hard at getting better to only end up feeling worse.

Here's how Trish will know the Dampness Reset is working:

- Feeling lighter, with stronger digestion and less bloating
- Clearer mind
- Increased energy
- Slow, steady weight loss
- Periods less heavy and more regular
- Fewer flareups of edema and skin rashes

Goals for Draining Dampness

You are about to undergo a metamorphosis. You'll emerge from the chrysalis feeling light and clear-headed, with subtle – maybe even dramatic – positive changes in your body and mind.

- Greater energy and mental clarity – imagine the fog lifting
- Slow, steady improvement in digestion and hormonal balance
- Growing ease and optimism about your life and health – a feeling that change is possible

Yes, Dampness is complex. But we'll get you set up with the tools you need to figure out what works and what doesn't work for your body.

Here's the key to the whole shebang: we're asking you to take the risk of putting YOU first. This will probably feel uncomfortable, but we believe you're up for it.

This means you'll need to start an exercise program – but don't panic! There's just one main exercise: building up your NO muscle so you can start saying YES to yourself.

What does YES look like? Well, for example, book in at least one relaxing Swedish or lymphatic draining massage. Start paying weekly visits to your local infrared sauna spa. Take five minutes each day to dry-brush your skin (see page 31). Get the idea?

These regular acts of self-love combined with powerful Damp-draining foods will soon have you slipping off your cocoon and taking flight.

Kitchen Medicine for Draining Dampness

We admit it: the Damp-reducing Reset is not the absolute MOST fun of the Yin Yang Resets.

But do you know what IS fun? Getting that bounce back in your step. Being able to digest your food and get fully nourished and energized so you can live and love your life again (or maybe even for the first time).

Ready to rumble? Here are the key words for reducing Damp:

- Light and simple
- Bitter
- Pungent

Eating simple meals of fresh veggies, lean meats, and whole grains means you'll no longer be creating Dampness. Instead, you'll be bathing your cells in nutrients while moving the old gunk out.

When we talk about eating simply, we do NOT mean deprivation. Hell no, we love food too much to go down that road. Picture, for example, a tasty fillet of grilled white fish with a squeeze of lemon and a sprinkle of fresh herbs served over a heap of fluffy basmati rice and mixed sautéed greens. Yummers.

The idea is to avoid overeating foods that are overly sweet, rich, fatty, and cold: sugary desserts, dairy, fatty meats, eggs, and an excess of raw salad and veggies.

What's that you say? Those are the very foods you crave?

We feel your pain. Would it help to know that, from a Western perspective, you may well have candida, a yeast overgrowth? Taking multiple rounds of antibiotics may have increased the likelihood for candida overgrowth. But whatever the cause of your cravings, feeding them perpetuates the storage of gunk, leading to Dampness imbalance … leading to more cravings.

Let's pause a moment and address these cravings. First of all, you are not alone. When you find yourself jonesing for sweets, check in with your body and ask if there's a deeper longing. Could it be that you really need a hug or you long to be truly heard? Before you dish up that bowl of ice cream, we invite you to give a friend a call. They want to hear from you, and opening yourself to care and support is a vital part of saying YES to yourself.

Okay, back to the food. We've talked about what to avoid. But what DO you eat?

The Dampness food chart arms you with powerful Damp-reducing foods. Traditional Chinese food therapy describes these foods as bitter, draining, and pungent.

Think bitter foods like dandelion, celery, and amaranth. Draining foods such as adzuki beans, alfalfa sprouts, and corn help dry up excessive fluids in the body. And pungent foods like mustard, horseradish, and onions are excellent for clearing out the stubborn sludge.

If you want a magical cure for Damp, you can't do better than bitters. Taking bitters (such as Swedish bitters) before meals naturally stimulates the production of saliva, gastric juices, and bile to prime your digestion. Bitters stimulate your appetite, prevent nausea and bloating, and help ease bowel discomfort.

Bitters not only signal the brain and stomach to prepare for the coming meal, they help repair that severed gut-brain connection. We recommend taking bitters before every meal so you can fully absorb the healing properties of your food. You'll still need to strictly adhere to the Dampness food chart, but we can confidently say you'll soon be feeling more like yourself. No wonder bitters have been around since the dawn of time!

A Word of Warning about Damp-Draining Foods

While bitters and other Damp-draining foods are hugely therapeutic, there's an art to using them. If your digestion is impaired (as it often is with Damp), you can make things worse by starting with too many Damp-drainers.

Remember, keep your diet light. Less is definitely more. Fewer ingredients prepared simply make digestion easier and help rebuild that crucial gut-brain connection. You could compare the Damp-reducing diet to when we introduce foods to an infant. Ideally, we start with single foods that are easy to digest. So go on, baby yourself!

If you're out for dinner, treat rich foods like condiments instead of main dishes. For example, if meat is served, take a small portion, then load up on lighter options, like grilled veggies.

What about treats? Well, in line with our anti-deprivation stand, you can enjoy a couple pieces of dark chocolate, as long as it's at least 80 percent cocoa, organic, and dairy free. Another Damp-reducing option is a little organic crystalized ginger. And we do mean a little. Beware of that fine line between treating yourself and overindulging. Take your time and really savour these healing treats. Let that chocolate melt in your mouth. You're welcome. :)

These Reset recipes will get you draining Dampness so your mind and body can feel vibrant and clear again. As you experiment with them, you'll start to notice what works for you and what doesn't. This self-awareness is key because the more you notice how food affects you, the more control you have over your health. We want you to put on a detective cap and investigate how you respond to the foods you eat.

That awareness will set you up for when you're back to your regular diet. If Damp symptoms start to flare again, you'll know what foods to add (and avoid) to get back on track.

Getting Started with the Dampness Reset

Dampness may be tricky, but it's no match for the Yin Yang Reset. We've devised a clear, simple plan of action for you.

We'll say it again: The secret to draining Dampness lies in the fine arts of simplicity and self-awareness. The foods you'll be eating over the next few weeks are primarily bitter and pungent. These qualities trigger your brain to release the enzymes and acids your gut needs to digest and absorb your food. As an added bonus, Damp-reducing foods also help curb your cravings.

Soon, you'll get the hang of picking Damp-moving foods and modifying your favourite recipes to include them.

And, hey, we'll tell you right now that Damp will NOT go down without a fight. So, if your mouth sometimes wins out over your brain in choosing what to eat, well, no shame, no blame. We've been there too. You've got what it takes to make positive changes - including super-delicious Damp-reducing recipes designed to win over your taste buds.

Now, go call someone who will hold you accountable because we want to see you succeed, and so does everyone around you. No more mud to trudge through, just clear skies and the easeful spreading of your beautiful wings.

Activities for Draining Dampness

Dampness needs purging so you need more vigorous activities. The goal is to burn up that excess by breaking a sweat.

Okay, we know: vigorous movement is probably the last thing you feel like doing. This resistance is normal when you have Dampness. If you can bust this open by moving at least three times a week, you'll give a serious boost to your healing. Great movement options for Dampness include:

- Walking and hiking
- Yoga, especially kinds that make you sweat, like hot yoga
- Running and other aerobic activities
- Cycling
- Sports
- Dancing

Try visiting an infrared sauna weekly as well. It's a wonderful treat that's relaxing, detoxing, beautifying for your skin, and great for stimulating a deep sweat and weight loss.

Beverages for Draining Dampness

Bitters – Swedish Bitters and Flora Gallexier Herbal Bitters. Take daily, before meals (follow directions on the label).

Dark Chocolate (80 percent or higher) – Enjoy up to 1 ounce (30 grams) as a treat 3 or 4 days per week. Make sure it's organic, with no milk ingredients.

Herbal coffee – Dandy Blend (we love this coffee substitute)

Medicinal teas – See "How to make medicinal teas" on page 61. Traditional Medicinals have some great Dampness-draining teas:

- Nettle
- Ginger
- Roasted Dandelion Root
- Burdock with Nettle
- Chamomile
- Ginger with Chamomile

Also try Organic India Tulsi Teas:

- Tulsi Chai (Holy Basil)
- Tulsi Turmeric Ginger (Holy Basil)

Dampness Reset Food Chart

Fruits	Vegetables	Grains
Berries	Broccoli	Amaranth
Lemon	Brussels sprouts	Buckwheat
Lime	Cabbage	Job's tears
Orange peel/zest	Carrots	Quinoa
Organic papaya	Chives	Rice
Pineapple	Daikon	Rye
	Garlic	
	Kohlrabi	**Herbs**
	Leafy greens	
	Leeks	Basil
	Mushrooms	Bay leaf
	Mustard greens	Cardamon
	Onions	Cinnamon
	Organic celery	Coriander
	Organic corn	Ginger
	Parsnips	Oregano
	Pumpkin	Rosemary
	Radish	Sage
	Rutabaga	
	Sprouts	
	Turnip	

Organic Protein	Additional	Foods to Avoid
Adzuki beans	Extra virgin olive oil	Fried foods
Black beans	Flax oil	Limit fruits
Broad beans	Horseradish	Nuts (except unsalted pistachio)
Chicken	Mustard	Soy
Fish	Raw honey	Sugar
Pinto beans	Stevia	Too much raw food
Pistachios		Wheat
Turkey		Alcohol
		Bananas
		Beef
		Caffeine
		Cow dairy
		Eggs
		Fatty meats

Sample Damp-Draining Meal Plans

Day 1

Breakfast: Apple Carrot Cinnamon Muffins and a cup of Tulsi Turmeric Ginger tea
Snack: Trail mix of sunflower seeds, pumpkin seeds, dried papaya, dried blueberries
Lunch: Salmon Salad Sandwich
Snack: Small bowl sweet potato and parsnip chips
Dinner: Succulent Slow Cooker Chicken with Daikon Carrot Slaw

Day 2

Breakfast: Savoury Breakfast Polenta
Snack: Small bowl of mixed berries
Lunch: Broccoli Chicken Pasta
Snack: Apple Carrot Cinnamon Muffins and cup of Tulsi Chai tea
Dinner: White Bean Turkey Chili

More Snack Options

- Pumpkin Spice Bread and a cup of ginger tea
- Pineapple Ginger Green Smoothie
- Hummus and rice crackers
- Asian Barley & Exotic Mushroom Soup
- Hummus and sprouts on an endive leaf boat

Day 3

Breakfast: White Bean Turkey Chili
Snack: Unsalted pistachio nuts and a cup of Burdock with Nettle tea
Lunch: Lettuce wrap with baked chicken, quinoa, celery, grated carrot, drizzled with vinaigrette
Snack: 3 pieces of organic crystallized ginger
Dinner: Turkey Tacos with Fresh Papaya Salsa and Apple Blondie Brownies

Day 4

Breakfast: Apple Blondie Brownies and cup of Ginger with Chamomile tea
Snack: Leftover Papaya Salsa and organic tortilla chips
Lunch: Vietnamese Salad Rolls and a cup of Roasted Dandelion Root tea
Snack: Air-popped organic popcorn
Dinner: Wild Rice & Leek Stuffed Portobello Mushroom

More Snack Options

- Unsweetened applesauce with 1 tbsp ground flax seed and cinnamon
- Turkey slices and fresh basil leaves wrapped in lettuce leaves
- Celery sticks with sunflower seed butter

Damp-Draining Breakfasts

Apple Carrot Cinnamon Muffins

Testing, testing 1, 2, 3 …10. Creating a muffin recipe for the Damp diet was a strategic nightmare because we couldn't use the usual ingredients like eggs, milk, butter, and wheat. After a LOT of testing (be grateful you're not trying batches 1 and 3, they weren't so tasty), we think we've nailed it. These muffins have all the elements you need to wake up and warm your digestive system. Break your fast with them alongside a cup of tea or stash them in your bag for a snack on the go. The raw honey clears the sludge of Dampness while the rice flour, carrots, and cinnamon support your digestion.

Protein tip: To boost your protein, pair this with our Pineapple Ginger Green Smoothie on page 129.

Makes 1 dozen

Dry
- 1 cup brown rice flour
- 1 cup white rice flour
- 1½ teaspoons baking soda
- 1 teaspoon cinnamon
- ½ teaspoon salt

Wet
- ⅓ cup olive oil
- ½ cup raw honey
- 1½ cups unsweetened applesauce
- 2 tbsp ground chia
- 1 cup grated carrot

1. Preheat the oven to 350°F. Prepare a 12-cup muffin tin with large paper liners.
2. In a medium bowl, combine the dry ingredients.
3. In a large bowl, whisk together the oil and honey. Add the applesauce and combine well. Whisk in the ground chia. Stir in the grated carrot.
4. Slowly pour the dry ingredients into the wet and whisk until smooth.
5. Spoon the batter into the prepared muffin tin and bake for 25 to 35 minutes, until a knife inserted comes out clean. The muffins will still be moist, so give them a little time to cool and set up before you dig in.

Savoury Breakfast Polenta

Start your morning with this bowl of goodness, tweaked here to pull the plug on Dampness while warming up and healing your gut (thank you, mushrooms, corn, garlic, and chilies). This satisfying breakfast will become a go-to for those days when you need to sustain your energy throughout your day.

Protein tip: To meet your protein needs, top with some cooked leftover ground turkey or chicken breast.

Serves 4

- 1 tbsp olive oil
- 1 small onion, diced
- 1 cup diced mushrooms
- 1 clove garlic, minced
- pinch red chili flakes
- 3 cups organic chicken or vegetable broth
- 1 cup organic cornmeal (we use Bob's Red Mill Organic Polenta Corn Grits)
- ½ cup grated carrot
- ¼ cup minced parsley
- freshly ground black pepper

1. In a medium saucepan, heat the olive oil over medium heat and sauté the onion for about 3 minutes, until it begins to turn translucent. Add the mushrooms, garlic, and chili flakes and cook for another 5 minutes.

2. Pour in the broth and bring to a boil. Slowly whisk in the cornmeal and reduce the heat to low. Toss in the carrot and simmer for 5 minutes, stirring occasionally.
3. Remove from the heat and stir in the parsley. Cover the pot and let sit for a few
4. minutes.
5. Season with black pepper and serve.

Quinoa & Red Bean Breakfast Hash

You're not alone if you crave savory breakfasts over sweet ones. This favorite can easily do triple duty as breakfast, lunch, or dinner! Want breakfast on the table in under 15 minutes? Use canned beans (we like Eden Foods brand) to cut down on cooking time. Whatever you do, don't sub in other beans. Adzukis are highly effective at draining away Dampness, so be sure to use them in this dish.

Ingredient tip: Yellow zucchini is easiest to find in summer and fall, when it's in season. If you can't find it, just substitute green zucchini.

Serves 4

- » 1 small onion, diced
- » 1 tbsp olive oil
- » 1 organic yellow zucchini, diced
- » ¾ cup grated carrots (about 3 carrots)
- » 4 green onions, sliced
- » ¼ cup minced fresh basil
- » 1 tsp dried oregano
- » ½ tsp salt
- » freshly ground black pepper
- » 2 cups cooked adzuki beans
- » 2 cups cooked quinoa

1. In a large frying pan over medium heat, sauté the onion in the olive oil until soft and translucent, about 5 to 7 minutes.

2. Add the zucchini, carrots, green onions, basil, and oregano. Season with salt and pepper. Cook for 3 to 5 minutes.
3. Stir in the cooked adzuki beans and quinoa, combine well, and heat until warmed through. Serve and enjoy.

Pineapple Ginger Green Smoothie

This makes a great quick breakfast or snack. Be sure to drink it at room temperature to protect your digestive "fire." Consuming cold smoothies can impair digestion, so warm it up. Using ginger and drinking this at room temperature will protect your digestion and help you better assimilate the nutrients. To get all the deets on using smoothies as part of your healing, see page 49.

Serves 1

- » 1 cup fresh or frozen pineapple chunks
- » 1 small handful organic kale (about ½ cup), stems removed and roughly chopped
- » ¼–½ inch piece ginger root, skin on
- » 2-3 cups room-temperature water or pure coconut water
- » 1 scoop protein powder

1. Place all ingredients in a high-powered blender and blend on high for 30 seconds, or until smooth and well combined.
2. Pour into a glass and bring to room temperature before consuming, if some of your ingredients were cold.

Damp-Draining Lunches

Salmon Salad Sandwich

Quick and easy, this classic is sure to satisfy your lunchtime hunger. If coworkers tease you for your "fishwich," it just means they're jealous. Let them eat their health-depleting fast food while nature's own medicine is putting you on the fast track to vibrant health.

Ingredient tip: For a light lunch, skip the bread and eat the salmon salad wrapped in a lettuce leaf.

Serves 2-3

- 1 can wild salmon, drained (we like Raincoast Trading)
- 1 stalk organic celery, finely diced
- 2 tbsp finely diced red onion
- ¼ cup loosely packed minced parsley
- 2-3 radishes, finely diced (about 2 tbsp)
- ¼ tsp salt
- freshly ground black pepper, to taste

Dressing
- 1 tbsp grainy mustard
- juice of ½ lemon

For serving
- lettuce
- gluten-free bread

1. In a small bowl, roughly break up the salmon with a fork. Add the celery, red onion, parsley, radishes, and salt and pepper to taste, mixing thoroughly.
2. Combine the dressing ingredients and toss into the salmon mix, combining well.
3. Heap lots of lettuce and a big scoop of salmon salad between two pieces of gluten-free bread and chow down.

Vietnamese Salad Rolls

These rolls are the BEST. They'll be your new food craving. Your first attempts at rolling the wraps might look like an Instagram fail, but have faith. You'll find the filling sweet spot to make these not only delicious, but photo-worthy. They're super-portable for meals at work or on the run. Using rice paper wraps and aromatic herbs keeps the meal light and easy to digest, putting a stop to the afternoon slump. The dip plays a vital role here, as the ginger (and chili, if using) adds extra digestive oomph.

Ingredient tip: Coconut aminos is a delicious soy alternative. You can find it at most health food stores or online.
Storage tip: Cover the rolls with damp unbleached paper towels to keep them fresh all day long.

Makes 12 rolls

Filling
- » 3-4 bunches vermicelli noodles (we use green bean thread LongKou noodles)
- » 5-6 carrots, grated
- » 2 cups shredded lettuce
- » 1 red bell pepper, sliced into thin strips
- » 1 bunch green onions, tops and bottoms trimmed, cut in half lengthwise
- » 24 fresh basil leaves

Optional additional fillings
- 1 papaya, thinly sliced
- 1 kohlrabi, peeled and cut into long, thin slices
- 1 yam, baked and cut into strips

Dipping sauce
- ½ cup coconut aminos
- 3 tbsp rice vinegar
- 1 tsp grated ginger root
- 1 tsp sesame oil
- a dash of chili paste, if you like it spicy
- 12 round rice paper wrappers

1. Bring a large pot of water to a boil. Add the vermicelli noodles and stir. Cook until noodles are al dente, about 2 to 3 minutes. Drain, rinse, and set aside.
2. Prepare all the other fillings and have on hand alongside the noodles.
3. To prepare the dipping sauce, in a small bowl whisk together all the ingredients.
4. To assemble, fill a large pan with hot water (we use a pie plate). Place 1 rice paper wrapper into the water, allow it to soften for about 10 seconds, then lift it out and hold it up for a few seconds to let the water drain off. Lay the wrapper on a damp kitchen towel to absorb excess water and hold it in place while you fill it.

5. Across the middle of the wrap, place a small handful of noodles, a bit of the vegetable filling, and a couple of basil leaves. Fold the bottom of the wrap up over the filling, then fold the two sides in and roll it up. The wrapper will be very sticky, so it will hold together well.
6. Repeat the process with the remaining wraps. Covering the wraps with a damp cloth will keep them fresh and moist for about a day at room temperature (though we doubt they'll last that long).

Broccoli Chicken Pasta Salad

Nearly every ingredient in this recipe is excellent at clearing Dampness, so go ahead and put this on weekly repeat.

Serves 4

- » 4 cups uncooked brown rice pasta spirals (we like Rizopia and Tinkyada brands)
- » 3 tbsp olive oil
- » 2 cloves garlic, minced
- » ¼ tsp chili flakes (optional)
- » zest of 1 lemon
- » ¼ cup minced parsley
- » 4 cups organic baby kale
- » 4 cups broccoli florets, steamed
- » 1-2 organic cooked chicken breasts, diced
- » juice of 1 lemon
- » salt and freshly ground black pepper, to taste

1. Cook the pasta according to package directions (about 7 to 10 minutes). Drain and rinse to cool the pasta and remove some of the starch. Place in a large bowl and set aside.
2. In a large frying pan, heat the olive oil over medium-low and sauté the garlic, chili flakes, and lemon zest for a minute.
3. Add the parsley and kale and continue to cook, stirring, until the kale becomes soft and wilted.
4. Toss in the broccoli and chicken, combining well.

5. Add the pan mixture to the cooked pasta bowl. Pour in the lemon juice and season with salt and pepper to taste. You might want to add extra lemon juice. Serve warm, or chill and enjoy as a cold salad.

Asian Barley & Exotic Mushroom Soup

This soup takes minutes to prepare and fills the house with a comforting aroma. Asian barley is a gluten-free grain that isn't as starchy as barley, so it doesn't suck all the liquid out of the soup. This grain is king when it comes to healing Damp symptoms in the body.

Ingredient tip: Asian barley is also known as Job's tears and coix seed. You can source it online or at any Asian grocery store.

Serves 6

- 2 tbsp olive oil
- 1 large onion, diced
- 4 cloves garlic, minced
- 1 lb mushrooms (shiitake, portobello, oyster), coarsely chopped
- ½ tsp thyme
- 8 cups organic chicken (or vegetable) broth
- 3 carrots, chopped
- 1 cup Asian barley, rinsed well in a strainer
- 2 tbsp coconut aminos
- sea salt and freshly ground black pepper, to taste

1. Heat the olive oil in a large stock pot over medium heat. Sauté the onion and garlic in the oil until the onion begins to brown, about 8 to 10 minutes.
2. Add the mushrooms and thyme and continue cooking, stirring occasionally, until the mushrooms are soft and start to brown.

3. Add the broth, carrots, Asian barley, and coconut aminos and bring to a boil. Reduce the heat to a gentle simmer, cover the pot, and cook for 50 to 60 minutes, until the Asian barley is soft and tender. Season with salt and pepper.

Damp-Draining Dinners

White Bean Turkey Chili

You can enter your next local chili cook-off with this one, touting all its therapeutic benefits. The clean, light flavours will earn you the gold medal, but your real win will be the newfound clarity, focus, and pep in your step. The Damp busters here are turkey, beans, celery, corn, and spices.

Serves 4

- 1 tbsp olive oil
- 1 large onion, chopped
- 1 lb organic ground turkey
- 4 cloves garlic, minced
- ½ tsp cumin
- ½ tsp oregano
- 1½ tbsp chili powder
- 1-2 tsp salt (depending on whether your broth is salted)
- freshly ground black pepper, to taste
- 2 cups chicken broth
- 4 medium-large carrots, chopped
- 4 stalks organic celery, chopped
- 14-oz can organic navy beans
- 2 bay leaves
- 1 cup frozen organic corn

1. In a large pot over medium heat, warm the olive oil and sauté the onion for 5 to 6 minutes until soft and translucent. Add the ground turkey, break it up with a wooden spoon, and cook, stirring occasionally, until

the turkey is no longer pink, about 5 to 6 minutes. Add the garlic and spices and sauté for 30 seconds.
2. Add the broth, carrots, celery, beans, and bay leaves to the pot, bring to a boil, and simmer for 30 to 45 minutes or until the carrots and celery are tender. Add the corn 10 minutes before serving.

Carrot Sweet Potato Soup

Welcome to the world's most adaptable Damp-diminishing dinner – so good you'll want to eat it for breakfast! This vegan soup can be served four ways. Swap the sweet potatoes for cabbage, celeriac, or parsnips. Enjoy each one for its unique draining properties and change it up for variety. Either way, keep it on the menu for when you need a simple, nourishing meal. You could also hearty it up by adding any cooked grain from the food chart (page 116).

Protein tip: Add some beans, like adzuki or white beans, to the soup for blood sugar balancing.

Ingredient tip: If you prefer your food a little meatier, use chicken broth in place of the veg broth.

Serves 4

- » 2 tbsp olive oil
- » 1 small onion, chopped
- » 3 stalks organic celery, chopped (about 1 cup)
- » 10-12 carrots, chopped (about 6 cups)
- » 1 medium sweet potato, chopped (about 1 cup)
- » 6 cups organic vegetable broth
- » ½ cup minced fresh parsley
- » sea salt and freshly ground black pepper, to taste

1. In a large pot, heat the olive oil over medium heat and sauté the onion for 1 to 2 minutes, until translucent. Add the celery, carrots, and sweet potato and cook for another 5 minutes, stirring occasionally.

2. Add the broth and bring to a boil. Reduce the heat, cover the pot, and simmer for about 25 minutes, or until the vegetables are tender.
3. Remove from the heat and blend until smooth using an immersion blender or Vitamix.
4. Stir in the fresh parsley and season with salt and pepper. Careful with the salt if you used salted broth.

Turkey Tacos with Fresh Papaya Salsa

Who doesn't love tacos? They're a treat to eat and simple to make. This salsa isn't only delicious, it's healing too. Sweet and bitter in flavour, papaya is the perfect digestive aid for reducing indigestion and congestion. You'll be dancing the papaya salsa all night long!

Serves 4

Taco filling
- » 1 tbsp olive oil
- » 1 lb organic ground turkey
- » ½ red onion, diced
- » 1 garlic clove, minced
- » 1½ tsp ground cumin
- » 2 tsp ground coriander
- » 1 tsp sea salt
- » freshly ground black pepper

Papaya salsa
- » 1 organic papaya, skinned, seeded, and diced into ¼-inch cubes
- » ¼ cup minced red onion
- » ¼ cup minced cilantro
- » pinch red pepper flakes
- » 2 tbsp lime juice
- » 8-12 organic corn tacos
- » 1 cup very thinly sliced green cabbage (about ¼ small head)

1. Preheat the oven to 350°F.
2. In a large frying pan, heat the olive oil over medium heat, and sauté the onion and garlic until the onion is translucent.
3. Add the ground turkey to the pan, breaking it up and browning. Sprinkle on the cumin, coriander, salt, and pepper, and cook for another 5 to 10 minutes or until the meat is cooked through.
4. Meanwhile, make the salsa. In a small bowl, combine all the ingredients and toss together.
5. Pop the tacos in the oven and warm them for a minute or two, until they're soft and chewy (but not crispy).
6. Scoop some turkey filling onto each taco and top with the thinly sliced cabbage and a heaping serving of papaya salsa. Yum!

Wild Rice & Leek Stuffed Portobello Mushrooms

Say hello to your new go-to dinner, as easy to make after a long day at work as it is nourishing. The key here is the fresh herbs. Their healing properties are bar none – the very essence of healing with whole foods. The mushrooms hold all the nourishing properties that will have your body naturally eliminating the toxins it's been hoarding. Mwah! You're welcome.

Preparation tip: Speed up your dinner prep by having the cooked rice on hand.

Serves 4

- ½ cup wild rice medley (we use Lundberg Wild Blend Rice)
- 1 cup chicken (or vegetable) broth
- 1 tbsp olive oil
- 2 leeks, white parts only, thinly sliced
- 2 cloves garlic, minced
- 2 stalks celery, finely chopped
- 1 tbsp minced fresh sage (or 1 tsp dried)
- 1 tbsp minced fresh rosemary (or 1 tsp dried)
- ½–1 tsp sea salt
- freshly ground black pepper
- 4 cups thinly sliced organic black kale (about 1 bunch)
- 4 portobello mushroom caps, wiped clean and stems removed

1. Cook the wild rice mixture according to package directions, using chicken stock instead of water to allow the rice to soak up the flavour.
2. Heat the oil in a frying pan over medium heat and sauté the leeks for 2 minutes, until they've softened. Add the garlic, celery, and seasonings. Reduce the heat to medium–low and cook for about 10 minutes, stirring occasionally.
3. Preheat the oven to 400°F.
4. Add the kale to the pan and cook, stirring occasionally, for another 10 minutes, until the kale is soft.
5. Remove from the heat, add the cooked rice, and combine well. Taste and adjust seasonings, if necessary.
6. Fill a 9 by 13-inch glass baking dish with ½ inch of water. Place the portobello caps in the dish (upside down) and spoon some filling into each cap.
7. Bake uncovered for 20 to 30 minutes, until the mushroom caps look slightly shriveled, the filling is lightly browned, and your kitchen is filled with a succulent 'shroomy aroma!

Lemon Basil Halibut

Treat yourself tonight and head to your local fish market for some fresh fish. While we suggest baking this in the oven, it's extra delicious grilled on the BBQ. Change it up by experimenting with the herbs listed in the Food Chart (page 116). The melt-in-your-mouth quality of this dish will make you proud to serve it to dinner guests.

Serving tip: Dish this up with oven-roasted asparagus and a steaming dollop of fluffy quinoa.

Serves 4

- 1-lb halibut fillet (or other firm white fish), cut into 2 pieces
- sea salt and freshly ground black pepper, to taste
- 1 tbsp olive oil
- 1 garlic clove, minced
- juice and zest of ½ lemon (top yellow skin only, not bitter white part underneath)
- ¼ cup chopped fresh basil

1. Rinse the fish under cool water and pat dry. Season with salt and pepper and place skin-side down in a small glass baking dish.
2. In a small bowl, combine the remaining ingredients. Pour over the fish and marinate, covered, for at least 30 minutes.
3. Preheat the oven to 400°F.
4. Bake the halibut in its marinade, uncovered, for 12 to 15 minutes, until it flakes easily with a fork.

Succulent Slow-Cooker Chicken with Daikon Carrot Slaw

Hands down, this flavour-bursting dish is our favourite! You can throw the ingredients into the pot in a mere 5 minutes, and it'll leave you feeling amazing. The wildly therapeutic daikon slaw aids digestion and helps avoid heaviness and bloat. Serve over cooked quinoa with a side of sautéed mustard greens.

Serves 4

Slow-cooker chicken
- » 1 tbsp olive oil
- » 2 cups chicken broth
- » 1 onion, diced
- » 2 cloves garlic, minced
- » 1 tsp ground cumin
- » 1 tsp chili powder
- » ½ tsp ground coriander
- » 1½ tsp sea salt
- » 1½ lb organic chicken breasts, boneless and skinless

Daikon carrot slaw
- » 2 tbsp lime juice
- » 2 tsp coconut aminos
- » 1 tsp raw honey (must be raw, to help eliminate Dampness from the body)
- » 1 cup grated carrots (about 3)

» 1 cup grated daikon

For serving
» cooked quinoa
» ¼ cup minced cilantro

1. For the chicken, combine all ingredients except the chicken in a slow cooker on low heat. Add the chicken breasts and toss to coat. Put on the lid and cook for 6 hours.
2. When the chicken is falling apart, shred the breasts with a fork and mix into the sauce.
3. For the slaw, in a medium bowl whisk together the lime juice, coconut aminos, and honey. Add the grated carrots and daikon and toss together.
4. To serve, scoop the shredded chicken onto hot cooked quinoa. Top with the daikon carrot slaw and sprinkle with cilantro.

Adzuki Bean & Squash Soup with Yummy Veggies

We've said it once, we've said it twice, and we'll just keep saying it: ADZUKI beans! This soup is warm and comforting to body and soul. When pumpkins are in season, use in place of the butternut. They're also excellent at removing Dampness and healing the body. Spice this soup up to your heart's content using the food chart (page 116). We've gotten rave reviews from a two-and-a-half year old, who asked for seconds and requested the soup again a week later!

Meal-planning tip: Double or triple this and freeze extra, pulling it out on nights when you're pressed for time.

Serves 4-6

- 1 cup uncooked adzuki beans, soaked 8 hours or overnight in 4 cups of water
- 1 tbsp olive oil
- 1 medium onion, diced
- 3 stalks celery, diced
- 1-2 tsp minced ginger root
- 2-lb butternut squash, peeled and diced into 1-inch cubes (about 4 cups)
- 6 cups organic chicken (or vegetable) broth
- 3 cups broccoli florets (about 1 large head)
- ½ cup frozen corn kernels
- 1 tsp salt

1. Put those adzukis on to soak at least 8 hours ahead of time.
2. In a large pot, heat the olive oil over medium heat. Sauté the onion for 2 to 3 minutes, until translucent. Stir in the celery and ginger and cook for another minute.
3. Drain and rinse the soaked adzuki beans. Add them to the pot along with the squash and broth. Bring to a boil, reduce to a simmer, cover, and cook for one hour, stirring occasionally.
4. Once the beans are soft, add the broccoli, corn, and salt and cook for 5 minutes.

Damp-Draining Desserts

Apple Blondie Brownies

Let's take a moment to bask in the glory of Yin & Yang, white & black, blondie & brownie (no blonde jokes here). While made with beans, these blondies have a rich caramel flavour profile with a marshmallowy texture from the dehydrated apples. While everyone is still on the black bean brownie bandwagon, you'll be rollin' into the next dinner party on the culinary cutting edge. These beanie little crowd pleasers are so damn healthy you can even eat them for breakfast sans guilt.

Makes 8–10

Batter
- 14-oz can organic navy beans (or any white bean)
- ½ cup + 2 tbsp rolled oats
- ¼ cup virgin coconut oil, melted
- ½ cup raw organic honey
- 2 tsp pure vanilla extract
- ½ tsp baking powder
- ½ tsp baking soda
- ¼ tsp salt

Topping
- ½ cup organic dehydrated soft apple pieces, minced into ¼-inch pieces

1. Preheat the oven to 350°F. Grease an 8 by 8-inch glass baking dish with coconut oil.

2. Combine all the batter ingredients in a food processor and blend for about 1 to 2 minutes. Don't worry if some oats are not entirely ground up, just blend until the batter is very smooth.
3. Pour the batter into the prepared pan and sprinkle the apple pieces on top. Bake for 25 minutes, until it starts to turn golden brown.
4. Allow to cool completely before cutting. Enjoy!

Pumpkin Spice Bread

Treat yourself to this spiced pumpkin bread with a hot cup of chai tulsi tea. The pumpkin and spices are amazing at drying Dampness. However, it's still a dessert, so don't indulge too often. We speak from experience, having eaten too much of this amazing bread in one sitting and paid for it. Take your bitters before that second slice. Temptation, she's a bitch!

Makes 1 loaf

Dry
- 1 cup brown rice flour
- ¾ cup tapioca flour
- 2 tbsp chia seeds, ground in a coffee grinder or Vitamix
- 1 tsp ground cinnamon
- ½ tsp ground ginger
- ½ tsp ground nutmeg
- ¼ tsp ground cloves
- 1 tsp baking powder
- ½ tsp baking soda
- ½ tsp sea salt

Wet
- 1 cup organic pumpkin purée
- ⅓ cup organic virgin coconut oil, melted
- ½ cup raw honey
- 4 tbsp water

1. Preheat the oven to 350°F. Grease a 9 by 5-inch loaf pan with coconut oil.
2. In a medium bowl, combine the dry ingredients.
3. In a large bowl, whisk together the wet ingredients.
4. Gently fold the dry mixture into the wet just until the dough is thick.
5. Pour into the prepared pan and bake for 45 to 50 minutes, or until the top is browned and a knife inserted into the centre comes out clean.
6. Cool in the pan for about 20 minutes. Gently remove to a rack and cool thoroughly before slicing.

Qi Deficiency Reset

What's Happening in Your Body when Your Qi Is Deficient?

Let's face it, you've lost your sparkle. Your energy is at an all-time low and brain fog rolls in at the most inconvenient moments.

Your meals are followed by a symphony of gas and burping, and you get so bloated that you end up bursting out of your pants – the ones that fit you this morning! And, in spite of digestive discomfort, you find it hard to stop eating. Surely a nice, rich dessert will perk you up, no?

You might be using up all your sick days and vacation in winter, and you've still got Kleenex tucked up your sleeve because you can't shake those sniffles. You may even burst into a sweat for no reason, like when you're walking down the stairs! You might even find yourself a little short of breath.

In Traditional Chinese Medicine this sparkle-depleted health pattern is called Qi Deficiency. It's often the early stage of the body going out of balance. Qi (say chee) is energy, vitality, and so much more. Depleted Qi means you don't have enough energy to efficiently digest your food. You don't even have the energy to know when you need to stop and chill out. Your body is crying out for deep nourishment.

What gives? Well, two things. First, your chore-to-rest ratio is off. Too much work, people. Not enough play and downtime.

And second, your food choices are tamping down your digestive "fire." Qi-depleting choices include too many processed snacks and those quick, "healthy" foods you eat to balance out the junk food, like ice-cold smoothies and raw salads.

Turns out those raw, cold foods are a recipe for Qi Deficiency. Think of your stomach as a cauldron where your digestive fire "cooks" the foods you eat and drink, breaking them down so you can absorb the nutrients. Ice-cold foods and beverages douse that fire. This slows your digestion and leaves particles of food undigested, leaving you starved for the nutrients and energy needed to build more Qi.

What Qi Deficiency can look like

Ashley wakes up with a flat tummy, but by evening she's popping out of her pants. She feels like she's got a lot of food sensitivities because so many foods make her bloated. We're talking gas of the epic variety. And as if that's not enough, she also suffers from loose bowel movements or diarrhea. A couple of practitioners have told her she probably has IBS.

Here are the signs that Ashley needs the Qi Deficiency Reset:

- Chronic digestive issues
- Easily fatigued
- Craving sweets
- Big-time overthinking and worrying
- Weak immune system that has her catching every cold

Ashley gets discouraged because even eating what she thinks is a "healthy" salad can make her belly blow up. On top of her daily digestive issues, her gut tends to purge when she gets nervous.

Here's how Ashley will know the Qi Deficiency Reset is working for her:

- Improved digestion, with no more bloating, gas, or discomfort after meals
- More energy
- Stronger immune system, so catching fewer colds
- Mentally grounded and at ease

Goals for Building Qi

Qi is not like the energy you get from drinking an espresso. Instead of the blowback of panic, anxiety, and jitters caused by overstimulation, abundant Qi will lead to:

- Stronger digestion and absorption of nutrients

- More grounded and relaxed, with balanced energy
- More robust immune system

You're here because your body is crashing, and we're asking you to perform CPR on yourself. How do you do that? It's simple (though not easy): Get in the habit of tuning in and taking action based on what you're noticing. In other words, learn to stop, look, listen – and act. Remember when you were little and you had endless energy to run and play all day? That's what we're going for here, but with the adult ability to tune in and notice when you need to rest.

As you rebuild your Qi, you'll feel like you're getting recharged for the first time in months, or even years. This is a calm, rooted, feel-good energy, steady and dependable, with no caffeine-buzz crash. Your body will be strong enough to accomplish the tasks of the day. You'll no longer feel like you're slogging uphill weighed down with a wet blanket. And speaking of blankets, you won't get chilled as easily so you can leave that just-in-case sweater at home.

You'll feel energized mentally and emotionally too, more optimistic and at peace. The hamster wheel of worry will gradually quiet down. If you've been a Nosy Nelly using other people's lives as a distraction, take heart. If the social-media rabbit hole of perfectly curated lives has you feeling like an Instagram fail, this is just your Qi Deficiency alerting you to pay closer attention to your thoughts and habits. Now you'll know to listen.

With sufficient Qi, your meals won't end with bloating, gas, and burping. You'll have the "energy" or Qi to properly digest and absorb your food and you'll feel satiated without dessert.

Digesting and absorbing more efficiently means you'll make it through your day unbloated. No more busting out the yoga pants as soon as you get home from work. Now you can wear them strictly for comfort, not to set your tummy free. Sure, you'll still be tired at the end of a busy day, but you'll have enough energy to notice when it's time to go to bed.

Kitchen Medicine for Building Qi

We're going back to basics, right to the very first foods we feed babies. If you're not a parent, just think of the easiest-to-digest foods with the greatest amount of nourishment and energy. These are the foods for building a healthy, robust body and immune system at every age. Here are the key words for Qi-building foods:

- Slow
- Warm
- Sweet

Think warm, slow-cooked, naturally sweet foods like mashed sweet potatoes and slow-cooked oats with stewed apples. These Qi-building foods are soft and easy to digest, which is why they're the first solid foods used to nourish a child after mother's milk. But baby's not the only one who says yum to well-dressed rice porridge, savoury roast chicken, and bright orange squash. These foods are as gently strengthening for your gut as they are for a young tummy new to solids.

How your food is grown and prepared magnifies its healing power. Slow-cooked complex carbs like whole grains and legumes build Qi. So do plants harvested later in the growing season, like starchy root vegetables and squash. *For months, these plants store up the sun's energy and the soil's nutrients in the form of carbohydrates, making them powerful Qi builders.* Basically, they're Mother Earth's battery packs. When it comes to building Qi, slow food rocks, so think slow growing and slow cooking.

And whenever you can, buy organic. Since you're counting on the stored energy in your food to heal you, go for food that stores the most energy. If root veggies are grown with chemical fertilizers and sprayed with biocides and pesticides, they can't deliver all the nutrients found in their organic counterparts. If you can afford to, buy sustainably grown, organic food is one of the best investments you can make in your health.

Food also gathers healing energy when you prepare it with care. Maybe you've got a favourite childhood dish that never quite turns out like when your mother made it for you. Now it's your turn to be the momma, whatever gender you identify as, and infuse love and care into everything you make.

The slower and longer you cook your food, the more healing it is. So set your Instant Pot aside for now and pull out your slow cooker. It will fill your kitchen with a sumptuous aroma while it breaks down the nutrients in your soups and stews, making them easy to absorb and assimilate. Long, slow cooking is a priceless kitchen elixir for healing digestive issues like bloating, gas, low appetite, and loose bowels.

Since stoking your digestive fire will heal your gut, cold foods are not your friend right now. Bid at least a temporary adieu to frozen treats like ice cream, cold drinks, and ice-cold smoothies. While you're at it, cut back on salad and other raw fruits and veggies too. Keep that gut fire burning strong!

Lastly, eating sweet foods is important for rebuilding your Qi – but we don't mean sugar, candies, or pop. Those processed non-foods are designed to be excessively – even addictively – sweet. Not only will they cause a rapid spike in your blood sugar, they can damage your digestion and spoil your taste buds for the more subtle sweetness of whole foods. We're talking about naturally, mildly sweet foods like sweet rice, butternut squash, carrots, and corn. These foods energize your body in a sustainable way that boosts your Qi, unlike processed sweets.

Once you're back in balance, you can use the Qi Deficiency diet as your go-to when you're heading into or recovering from a cold or transitioning to a cooler, darker season. These meals will fill your home with aromas that trigger your parasympathetic nervous system, also known as your "rest and digest" mode.

Getting Started with Building Qi

We know, you've tried every single diet on the planet and nothing has worked ... yet. This is where we come in. The Yin Yang Reset is not something you'll stay on for the rest of your life. It's a temporary lifestyle shift you can come back to when you need a boost or just want to feel like yourself again.

You've probably felt defeated by all the time and effort you've spent transforming your kitchen into superfood central without results. How do we know this? Because we've been there too. We see you in the grocery lineup comparing what you're buying with the latest "health" foods in the Dr. Oz magazine. We'll even go out on a limb and say that your cart is full of salad and smoothie ingredients. And of course you've tossed in that little sugary treat, because you've earned it with all the so-called healthy food and, anyway, you can't get through the day without it.

We say forget the latest belly-and-bloat-busting fad. The ancient wisdom behind Traditional Chinese food therapy tells us that complex carbs in moderation, combined with specific Qi-building foods, are actually good for you.

So, put down that magazine and let Mother Earth serve up the exact nutrient-dense Qi-filled foods you need to recharge your battery. Say so long to bloat, endless colds, flagging energy, and maybe even your yoga pants.

Activities for Building Qi

When your Qi is deficient, your energy quickly flags, no matter how motivated you are to get yourself moving. If you manage to get out and run every day, you only last a week before you run out of steam. We get it: everything seems hard because you tire so easily.

But exercise is essential for your physical and emotional body, so what can you do?

Here's the plan. (You might notice that it's similar to the activity plan for Blood Deficiency, because the two imbalances share this low energy.) Start slowly and work up to moving at least three times a week. Remember, your key word for all activities is GENTLE. Your best bet for building Qi is low-intensity exercises that get your Qi moving. Aim for feeling energized but not exhausted. Here are some good options:

- Walking and hiking
- Gentle yoga, like hatha, restorative, and yin
- Gentle swimming
- Cycling
- Slow dancing with a partner
- Slow sports like badminton, ping-pong, and 9-hole golf

Extra points for taking these activities outside to harness the energy of nature. Even more points for bringing a friend along.

Meditation is also great for slowly building up Qi, so join a group or download an app, or get back to that practice you used to do — you know, the one that worked so well until you stopped doing it. For a daily 10-minute meditation, we like the Sam Harris Waking Up app.

We have one last prescription for you that's an unparalleled Qi-builder: hugs and cuddles. (You'll notice it's in the Blood-Building Reset too.) Put yourself in the path of love and fill up your love bucket every chance you get.

Beverages for Building Qi

Herbal coffee – Dandy Blend (we love this coffee substitute)

Herbal and medicinal teas – See "How to make medicinal teas" on page 61. Traditional Medicinals have some great Qi boosting teas:

- Ginger with chamomile
- Gingeraid
- Nettle leaf
- Fennel
- Roasted dandelion root

Also try Organic India Tulsi Teas:

- Tulsi licorice spice
- Tulsi chai

Qi Deficiency Reset Food Chart

Fruits	Vegetables	Grains
Cooked and dried fruits Cooked organic apples Dates Figs Orange peel/zest Organic cherries Organic grapes Organic strawberries	Arugula Carrots Garlic Green, red or savoy cabbage Leeks Mushrooms Onions Organic corn Organic potatoes Parsnips Peas (fresh or frozen) Pumpkin Rutabaga Sweet potatoes Turnips Winter squash Yams	Gluten-free oats Mochi Quinoa Rice Spelt Sweet rice **Herbs** Anise seed Basil Black pepper Caraway seeds Cayenne pepper Cinnamon Fennel seed Ginger Licorice root

*Butter is the only form of dairy in the Qi Deficiency Reset.

Organic Protein	Additional	Foods to Avoid
Anchovies Beef Black beans Chicken Chickpeas Halibut Lamb Mackerel Tuna Turkey Yellow split peas	Chestnuts Organic butter* Organic molasses Organic tomato paste**	Napa or Chinese cabbage Raw food Seaweed Spinach Sprouts Swiss chard Amaranth Bananas Dairy Fresh tomatoes Ice cold drinks, foods, smoothies Millet Mint
More Herbs		
Nutmeg Parsley Rosemary Star anise Thyme		

**Though tomatoes are not in this diet plan, we've used organic tomato paste in some of the recipes because it adds depth and flavour and is more easily digested, being the most cooked and warmed form of the tomato.

Sample Qi-Building Meal Plans

Day 1

Breakfast: Cinnamon-Currant Baked Oatmeal with a cup of Roasted Dandelion Root tea
Snack: Toasted gluten-free bread with butter and fig jam with a cup of Licorice Spice tea
Lunch: Chickpea "Tuna" Salad Sandwich
Snack: Organic corn tortilla chips and guacamole
Dinner: Savoury Shepherd's Pie

Day 2

Breakfast: Savoury Shepherd's Pie
Snack: Granola clusters and coconut yogurt with a cup of Tulsi Chai tea
Lunch: Honey Lime Sesame Salad in a Jar
Snack: Energy Balls: oats, almond butter, honey with dried apples and raisins with a cup of Ginger with Chamomile tea
Dinner: Kale, Mushroom, & Sweet Corn Congee

More Snack Options

- Vanilla Strawberry Apple Crisp
- Tuna salad on top of almond crackers
- Bowl of granola with coconut or almond milk

Day 3

Breakfast: Kale, Mushroom, & Sweet Corn Congee
Snack: Fruit medley: dried cherries, raisins, figs, and dates with a cup of Ginger with Chamomile tea
Lunch: Chickpea Hummus Platter
Snack: Apple Cinnamon Brown Rice Muffins with a cup of Nettle Leaf tea
Dinner: Zesty Cilantro Turkey Meatballs

Day 4

Breakfast: Strawberry Apple Pie Smoothie
Snack: Roasted chestnuts (we like the Dan-D-Pak Organic Chestnuts)
Lunch: Sesame Chicken Pasta Salad
Snack: Rice cakes/crackers with butter and cherry jam
Dinner: Yam Quesadillas with Walnut Basil Pesto

More Snack Options

- Mochi with a cup of Tulsi Chai tea
- Date square with a cup of Roasted Dandelion tea
- Vegan rice pudding
- Organic corn chips with hummus

Qi-Building Breakfasts

Strawberry Apple Pie Smoothie

Strawberries, apples, and pie ... OH, MY! Bet you never had a smoothie with cooked apples. Not only do the cooked ingredients make this smoothie unique, they're kinder to your gut, allowing it to heal. You can more easily absorb and assimilate your nutrients from cooked foods, and that boosts your Qi, which boosts your energy.

Digestion tip: Drink your smoothies at room temperature. In fact, avoid ALL cold drinks because they can dampen your digestive "fire." Eating room-temperature and warm cooked foods strengthens your gut and your health. (Get all the deets on using smoothies to heal over on page 49.)

Serves 1

- » ½ cup organic applesauce
- » ½ cup organic strawberries
- » 1 cup almond (or coconut) milk
- » 1-2 cups room temperature water (depending on how thick you like it)
- » 1 scoop protein powder (see page 48 for our favourites)
- » 1 tbsp ground flax seed
- » ½ tsp ground cinnamon

1. Combine all ingredients in a blender or Vitamix and blend for 30 seconds, or until smooth.

Apple Cinnamon Brown Rice Muffins

This beautiful, hearty, warm-your-soul muffin will have you coming back for more. Whether for breakfast, lunch, or snack, we dare you to eat just one! The healing properties of the rice flour, butter, and fragrant cinnamon are immune and Qi boosting, while the cooked apples make for strong, healthy digestion.

Protein tip: To meet your protein needs, pair with our Strawberry Apple Pie Smoothie on page 181.

Makes 10-12 muffins

Dry
- 1½ cups brown rice flour (we use Bob's Red Mill)
- ½ cup tapioca flour
- 2 tsp ground cinnamon
- 2 tsp baking powder
- ½ tsp baking soda
- ½ cup coconut palm (or organic) sugar
- 2 tbsp chia seeds, ground in a coffee grinder or Vitamix

Wet
- 2 eggs
- 1 ⅓ cups almond (or coconut) milk
- ⅓ cup melted organic butter
- 2 large organic apples, diced into small pieces
- ½ cup raisins (optional but delicious)

1. Preheat the oven to 350°F. Grease a 12-cup muffin tin with butter or coconut oil, or do what we do and line with paper cups.
2. In a medium bowl, stir together the dry ingredients thoroughly.
3. In a large bowl, beat the eggs. Whisk in the milk and melted butter.
4. Slowly add the dry ingredients into the wet, stirring after each addition. Gently fold in the apples and raisins, if using.
5. Pour the batter into the prepared muffin tin and bake for 30 minutes. A knife inserted in the centre may not come out perfectly clean because of the fruit. Don't worry, the muffins will firm up as they cool, so try not to eat them all at once!

Cinnamon-Currant Baked Oatmeal

There's something so satisfying about a bowl of piping-hot oatmeal in the morning. This breakfast casserole takes your childhood instant oatmeal to the next level. The oats are fluffy straight out of the oven and pair beautifully with a dollop of coconut yogurt. This also makes a great on-the-go snack. Just let it cool and cut it into squares to munch while you're out and about or simply standing over your kitchen sink.

Protein tip: To boost your protein needs, pair with our Strawberry Apple Pie Smoothie on page 181.

Serves 4

Dry
- 1½ cups quick-cooking rolled oats
- ¼ cup dried currants (or raisins)
- ¼ cup chopped walnuts
- 2 tsp cinnamon
- 1 tsp baking powder
- pinch sea salt
- 1 apple, cored and diced

Wet
- 1 organic egg
- 1 cup almond (or coconut) milk
- 2 tbsp avocado (or olive) oil
- ¼ cup honey
- coconut or almond yogurt (optional)

1. Preheat the oven to 375°F. Grease an 8 by 8-inch baking dish with butter or coconut oil.
2. In a medium bowl, combine the oats, currants, walnuts, cinnamon, baking powder, and salt. Mix in the diced apple.
3. In a small bowl, beat the egg and whisk in the milk, oil, and honey.
4. Pour the wet mixture into the dry and stir to combine.
5. Spread into the prepared baking dish and bake for 30 to 35 minutes, until the oatmeal looks set and has turned a golden brown.
6. Serve in bowls on its own or topped with a dollop of non-dairy yogurt.

Cauliflower Black Bean and Roasted Red Pepper Wraps

That's a wrap, folks! Honestly, what's not to love about wrapping up a meal! The Qi superfoods here (garlic, black beans, parsley, and tortillas) give you an authentic energy boost that will sustain you throughout your day.

Wrap tip: Try a variety of gluten-free wraps and find your favourite. We love coconut, cassava, almond flour, and dehydrated veggie wraps. Find them at your local health food store (often in the frozen foods).

Serves 4

- » 1 organic red pepper, roasted (or about 2 organic roasted red peppers from a jar)

Bean filling
- » 2 tbsp olive oil
- » 1 cup finely chopped cauliflower
- » 1 stalk organic celery, chopped
- » 1 clove garlic, minced
- » 14-oz can black beans (1½ cups cooked)
- » ½ tsp ground coriander
- » ½ tsp ground cumin
- » ½ tsp sea salt
- » freshly ground black pepper, to taste
- » 4 soft gluten-free tortillas
- » Optional toppings
- » 1 cup minced parsley
- » 4 green onions, thinly sliced

1. If you're roasting your own pepper, preheat the oven broiler. Place the whole pepper on a baking sheet and roast for 15 to 20 minutes. Turn the pepper every few minutes as the skin begins to blacken. Make sure to lightly blacken all sides. Remove from the oven, place the pepper in a bowl, and cover the bowl with a plate or plastic wrap to steam it. After about 10 minutes, peel the skin off, slice the pepper in half, scoop out the seeds, and slice it into long strips. Set aside.
2. To make the bean filling, heat the oil in a medium frying pan over medium heat and sauté the cauliflower and celery for 5 minutes. Add the garlic and cook for another minute. Pour in the black beans, sprinkle with the coriander, cumin, salt, and pepper, and sauté for another 3 to 5 minutes. Remove from the heat and mash to a chunky consistency with the back of a spoon.
3. For the tortillas, pop them into a 350°F oven and warm them for a minute or two, until they're soft and chewy (but not crisp).
4. To serve, spoon some bean filling into the middle of each tortilla and top with roasted red pepper slices, parsley, and chopped green onions. Roll up and chow down.

Qi-Building Lunches

Chickpea "Tuna" Salad Sandwich

As the chef, you'll now know what's going into your food. This dish is delicious, colourful, and filling, delightful for both vegans and old-school tuna lovers. Pack this up and you'll be the one in the lunchroom with the fresh new take on that same-old stinky-fish sammie.

Vegan tip: Make this plant-based by using a vegan mayonnaise like Vegenaise.

Wrap tip: If you want to lighten this up, try a gluten-free wrap instead of bread. We love coconut, cassava, almond flour, and dehydrated veggie wraps. Find them at your local health food store (often in the frozen foods).

Serves 4

Chickpea "tuna"
- » 14-oz can chickpeas (1½ cups)
- » 3-4 tbsp organic mayonnaise
- » 1½ tsp rice (or apple cider) vinegar
- » 1 tbsp Dijon mustard
- » ½ tsp ground turmeric
- » 1 stalk organic celery, finely diced
- » 1 tbsp finely diced red onion
- » ¼ cup minced parsley,
- » ¼ tsp sea salt
- » pinch cayenne pepper

For serving
- » gluten-free (or 100% spelt or oat) bread
- » mixed greens
- » 1 carrot, grated

1. In a medium bowl, roughly mash the chickpeas with the back of a spoon or a potato masher. You're going for chunky, not smooth.
2. Mix in the rest of the "tuna" ingredients until well combined.
3. To assemble, toast the bread (or warm the wraps), heap on the chickpea tuna, and top with mixed greens and grated carrot.

Honey Lime Sesame Salad in a Jar

Maybe you've seen them on Instagram and said, "come on, salad in a jar?" Well, once it's on your counter, it won't just be eye candy, it'll be positively mouth-watering. As a bonus you'll never feel bloated again after eating salad. Our secret? Cook your salads. Poof!

Digestion tip #1: Marinating your cabbage in a vinaigrette helps break down the raw, hard-to-digest bits. Keep the crunch, ditch the bloat and gas. But if cabbage is NOT your friend, you have two options: lightly sauté it before adding to the jar or simply leave it out. To make this without cabbage, assemble the remaining ingredients and toss with the dressing right before eating. Expecting leftovers? Reserve some of the salad and dressing in separate containers, and combine when you're ready to serve.

Digestion tip #2: To improve digestibility, serve with some hot, cooked meat like slow-cooker chicken, grilled halibut, or beef kabobs.

Serves 2 generously

Dressing
- ¼ cup olive oil
- 1 clove garlic, minced
- 1 tsp apple cider (or rice or wine) vinegar
- ½ tsp sesame oil
- juice of one lime
- 1 tbsp honey
- pinch sea salt
- freshly ground black pepper

Salad
- » 2 cups very thinly sliced red cabbage
- » 2 cups cooked quinoa
- » 1 large yam, baked and cut into cubes
- » 1½ cups organic corn kernels
- » 4 green onions, chopped
- » 4 cups mixed baby salad greens

1. Have two 1-quart Mason jars on hand.
2. In a small bowl, whisk together all the dressing ingredients.
3. Pour half the dressing into the bottom of each jar. Add half the cabbage so it can marinate in the dressing and prevent the rest of the salad from getting soggy. (Remember: no marinating if you're leaving out the cabbage, otherwise the greens will get soggy.)
4. Divide the remaining ingredients between the two jars in the order listed (quinoa, yams, corn, green onion, mixed baby greens) and refrigerate for at least 1 hour, preferably overnight.
5. When ready to serve, put in a bowl and toss the marinated cabbage and dressing evenly throughout the salad.

Chickpea Hummus Platter

Who wants first dip? Crudités are a mainstay in our homes — quick finger food for the littles and easy-to-grab grub for grown-ups on the go. Once the hummus is made, there's not much to this. Choose some Qi-friendly veggies for dipping, give them a quick steam (or blanch) to increase their digestibility, and you're off to the Qi-building races. You can prepare the veg in advance and store in the fridge to use with the hummus or to have on hand as a healthy snack.

Serves 4

Hummus
- 14-oz can chickpeas (1½ cups cooked)
- ¼ cup tahini (sesame seed paste)
- ½ cup water
- 2 cloves garlic, chopped
- ½ tsp ground cumin
- ½ tsp ground coriander
- ½–1 tsp sea salt
- juice of 1½ lemons
- ⅛–¼ tsp cayenne pepper (to taste)

Dipping options
- carrot sticks
- fennel wedges
- broccoli
- cauliflower
- organic corn tortilla chips

1. Combine all the hummus ingredients in a food processor and blend until smooth and creamy. If it's too thick, add more water.
2. Place your choice of dipping veggies in a steamer basket and steam for 3 minutes, or until crisp–tender.
3. Serve the hummus in a bowl with an assortment of crisp, steamed vegetables and a heap of corn chips.

Sesame Chicken Pasta Salad

One-dish wonder to the rescue! We, your fairy godmothers, have sprinkled a whole lotta sparkle into this bowl. Poof, dinner is served. Even better, enjoy this for lunch, or why not breakfast?! It's the chicken, carrots, corn, peas, and pasta that deliver the Qi power. They'll boost your energy AND take a load off your digestion.

Prep tip: For maximum flavour, give yourself an extra half hour at the end to let the pasta soak up the dressing.

Serves 4

Chicken
- » 2 organic chicken breasts
- » olive oil, for drizzling
- » salt and freshly ground black pepper

Dressing
- » 2 tbsp olive oil
- » ¼ cup tamari soy sauce (or Bragg Liquid Aminos)
- » ¼ cup rice vinegar
- » 1 tbsp maple syrup (or honey)
- » ½ tbsp toasted sesame oil

Pasta
- » 8 oz gluten-free corkscrew pasta (brown rice, corn, or quinoa)
- » ½ cup fresh or frozen organic corn kernels
- » ½ cup fresh or frozen organic peas
- » 2 carrots, grated
- » 4 green onions, chopped

1. Preheat the oven to 400°F.
2. Place the chicken breasts on a baking sheet and drizzle with olive oil and a pinch of salt and pepper. Bake for 20 to 25 minute, until cooked through.
3. Meanwhile, in a small bowl, whisk together the dressing ingredients and set aside.
4. Bring a medium pot of water to the boil and cook the pasta according to package directions, or until done to your liking (usually 7 to 10 minutes). Drain and rinse the pasta and place it in a large bowl.
5. Cut the chicken breasts into ½-inch cubes and toss into the pasta bowl along with the corn, peas, grated carrots, and green onions. (The heat of the pasta should thaw the frozen veg.)
6. Pour ½ to ⅔ of the dressing onto the pasta, toss, and let the flavours meld for about 30 minutes before serving. You can add a little of the reserved dressing when you're ready to eat.

Qi-Building Dinners

Turmeric Ginger Noodle Soup

Turmeric is gold! The colour gold is amazing for building your Qi. You might want to go a little heavy handed on this spice for all its healing powers, and we say do it. This warm and aromatic bowl of goodness is simple and very healing to your digestive system. It stands alone as a meal or makes a beautiful accompaniment to the Yam Quesadillas (page 205).

Noodle tip: Gluten-free pastas are starchy. For a clearer, consommé-style soup, cook the noodles separately and add them to each bowl before serving.

Serves 3

- 1 tbsp olive oil
- 1 small onion, diced
- 3 medium carrots, chopped into chunks
- 1 tsp peeled, minced ginger root
- 1 tsp ground turmeric
- 6 cups organic chicken (or vegetable) broth
- 1¼–1½ cups brown rice elbow pasta (we like Rizopia and Tinkyada brands)
- 4 cups finely chopped organic kale
- freshly ground black pepper

1. In a large saucepan, heat the olive oil over medium heat and sauté the onion for 3 minutes, until translucent. Add the carrots, ginger, and turmeric, and cook, stirring lots, for another 3 minutes.

2. Pour in the broth and bring to a boil. Add the noodles and cook until tender, about 7 to 10 minutes, depending on the kind you use.
3. Stir in the kale and immediately take the pan off the heat. Season with salt to taste and a few grinds of pepper, and serve.

Zesty Cilantro Turkey Meatballs

The unique flavour combination of soy, ginger, and cilantro makes this one of our favourite meals. So delicious and easy, why not whip up extra batches and freeze them to pull out for instant dinners? Garlic, ginger, and cilantro are the medicinal medley that will promote the healing force in your body and bring you back to Flat Stomach City.

Tip: If you want a lighter meal, substitute spaghetti squash for the pasta.

Serves 4

Meatballs
- » 1 lb ground organic turkey
- » 1 organic egg, beaten
- » 1 tbsp tamari soy sauce (or Bragg Liquid Aminos)
- » 1 tsp minced garlic
- » 1 tsp minced ginger root
- » ½-1 tsp ground cumin
- » ½ tsp chili pepper flakes (optional)
- » ¼ cup minced cilantro
- » ¼-⅓ cup gluten-free bread crumbs (use rice flour in a pinch)
- » 2 tbsp olive oil

Pasta
- » 1-lb package brown rice elbow pasta (we like Rizopia and Tinkyada brands)
- » 2 tbsp organic butter
- » 1 small onion, diced
- » 1 carrot, grated
- » 1 small organic zucchini, diced
- » salt and freshly ground black pepper, to taste

1. In a medium bowl, combine the turkey, egg, soy sauce, garlic, ginger, cumin, and chili flakes. Stir in the cilantro and bread crumbs. Roll into about 12 to 16 ping-pong-size balls.
2. In a large frying pan, heat the 2 tablespoons of olive oil over medium heat. Fry the meatballs until they are golden brown on all sides and cooked through. Set aside on a paper-towel-lined plate.
3. Cook the pasta according to package directions (about 7 to 10 minutes). Drain, rinse, and set aside.
4. Heat 2 tablespoons of butter in a large frying pan over medium heat, and sauté the onion until soft and translucent. Add the carrot and zucchini and cook for 3 to 5 minutes, until soft. Toss in the cooked brown rice noodles and season with salt and pepper.
5. To serve, scoop the buttered noodles and vegetables onto a plate and top with some hot meatballs.

Yam Quesadillas with Walnut Basil Pesto

The texture profile of sautéed onions, mashed yams, and roughly mashed beans is AMAZING. Don't be surprised if, after serving, you hear things like this around the table: "These are killer, I could eat them all day." You can thank Mother Earth for this one. Yams pull up their healing goodness from deep within the earth to build Qi in the mitochondria in each of your cells.

Wrap tip: Try a variety of gluten-free wraps and find your favourite. We love coconut, cassava, almond flour, and dehydrated veggie wraps. Find them at your local health food store (check the frozen foods).

Serves 4

- » 1 large yam

Walnut pesto
- » ¼ cup olive oil
- » 1½ cups fresh basil leaves
- » 1 clove garlic, chopped
- » juice of ½ lemon
- » ¼ cup + 1 tbsp walnut halves
- » ¼ tsp sea salt

Beans
- » 1 tbsp olive oil
- » 1 small onion, diced
- » 19-oz can black beans (2 cups cooked)
- » ¼ tsp sea salt
- » freshly ground black pepper, to taste
- » eight 8-inch soft tortillas, preferably rice or corn (we like Food for Life Brown Rice Tortillas)

1. Preheat the oven to 400°F.
2. Bake the yam for about 45 minutes, until fork tender. Scrape the yam meat off the skins and into a small bowl, and mash.
3. Combine all the pesto ingredients in a food processor and blend thoroughly. Set aside.
4. In a medium frying pan, heat the olive oil over medium heat and sauté the onion for 3 minutes. Mix in the black beans, salt, and pepper and cook for another 3 minutes. Remove from the heat and smash with a fork (but keep it chunky).
5. To assemble, spread the cooked yam all over 4 of the tortillas and top each with ¼ of the bean mixture. Place the remaining tortillas on top and squish them down so they stick together.
6. In a medium frying pan, heat a little butter or oil over medium heat. Cook the quesadillas on each side until lightly browned and crispy.
7. Cut into quarters and serve with the Walnut Pesto.

Kale, Mushroom, & Sweet Corn Congee

Welcome to the ultimate traditional Chinese food formula. Congee is long revered for its healing properties. Warm and easily digested, it nourishes and builds blood, Qi, and Yin. This dish could be dinner for breakfast, then for lunch. Show yourself even more love by doubling the recipe.

Topping tip: We enjoy our congee topped with a drizzle of soy sauce, some chili paste, and a few chopped green onions.

Serves 4

Congee
- 1 tbsp olive oil
- 1 large onion, diced
- 2 cloves garlic, minced
- 2 cups sliced mushrooms (cremini, oyster, button, enoki, shiitake, etc.)
- ⅔ cup jasmine rice
- 6 cups organic chicken (or vegetable) broth
- 1 cup organic corn kernels
- 4 leaves organic kale, chopped

Topping options
- tamari soy sauce (or Bragg Liquid Aminos)
- chopped green onions
- sambal chili paste
- freshly ground black pepper

1. In a large pot, heat the olive oil over medium heat and sauté the onion until translucent. Add the garlic and mushrooms and cook until the mushrooms are soft.
2. Stir in the rice, pour in the broth, and bring to a boil. Reduce the heat to a low simmer, cover, and cook for one hour, stirring occasionally.
3. Add the corn kernels and cook for another 20 minutes. Toss in the chopped kale and cook for 10 minutes longer.
4. Yum it up with your choice of toppings and serve.

Garlic Butter Mushrooms with Yellow Rice

Say hello to your new weekly 30-minute comfort dish. You'll be whistling and smiling as you sprinkle turmeric into your cooking rice. The aroma filling your kitchen will pull in the curious to ask what's for dinner. The earthy texture of the mushrooms combines with the butter and garlic to send your oxytocin levels up into their happy place.

Serves 4

Yellow rice
- 2 cups rice (jasmine and basmati are our favourites)
- 2-4 cups water (depending on type of rice)
- 1 tsp ground turmeric

Garlic butter mushrooms
- 1 tbsp olive oil
- 2 tbsp organic butter
- 6 cups sliced mushrooms (cremini, oyster, button, enoki, shiitake, etc.)
- 1 clove garlic, minced
- 6 cups chopped collard greens (or organic kale or bok choy)
- sea salt and freshly ground black pepper, to taste

1. In a medium saucepan, combine the rice, water, and turmeric and cook for about 15 minutes, or according to package directions.
2. Meanwhile, in a large frying pan, warm the olive oil and butter over medium heat, and sauté the mushrooms for about 5 minutes, until they begin to soften.
3. Add the garlic and chopped greens and cook for another 15 minutes, until the greens are soft and tender. Season to taste with salt and pepper.
4. Serve over the hot rice.

Savoury Shepherd's Pie

Do yourself a favour and make a double or triple batch because this super-Qi-healing recipe will keep everyone coming back for more. You'll be craving seconds, going back for thirds, and wishing you had leftovers for lunch tomorrow.

Freezer tip: This dish freezes and defrosts beautifully for a quick dinner during the week.

Serves 4-6

- 4 organic Yukon gold potatoes, chopped into 1-inch chunks
- 2 tbsp organic butter
- 1 tsp sea salt
- 1 tbsp olive oil
- 1 onion, diced
- 1 cup thinly sliced carrots
- 2 cups thinly sliced mushrooms (any variety)
- 1 tsp thyme
- 2 tsp rosemary
- 1 lb extra-lean organic ground beef
- freshly ground black pepper
- 1 tbsp organic tomato paste
- 1 tsp Worcestershire sauce (gluten-free, if possible)
- 1½ tbsp brown rice flour
- 1 cup organic beef bouillon
- ½ cup fresh or frozen organic peas

1. Preheat the oven to 400°F. Have an 8 by 8-inch baking dish on hand.
2. In a large saucepan, cover the potatoes with water and bring to a boil. Reduce the heat and simmer for 10 to 15 minutes, until fork tender.
3. Drain the potatoes and return to the pot. Add the butter and ½ teaspoon of the salt, and mash the potatoes until fluffy and well combined.
4. While the potatoes boil, heat the olive oil in a large frying pan over medium heat and sauté the onion for 2 minutes.
5. Add the carrots, mushrooms, thyme, and rosemary. Cook for another 3 minutes, just until the vegetables begin to soften.
6. Add the ground beef, remaining ½ teaspoon of salt, and some pepper, and cook for about 3 to 5 minutes, until the meat is browned.
7. Add the tomato paste and Worcestershire sauce. Sprinkle on the flour and stir it in. Add the beef bouillon, bring to a boil, reduce the heat, and simmer gently for 5 minutes, or until the mixture thickens. Stir in the peas.
8. Put the beef mixture into the baking dish and spread the mashed potatoes on top. Bake for 30 minutes.
9. Slice into squares, serve piping hot, and watch it disappear!

Mom's Nomato Beef Stew

This recipe holds a special place in our hearts. When the Yin Yang Reset team rocked up to the table with a laundry list of things we couldn't eat (like tomatoes), it was Mom to the rescue! She whipped out her Instant Pot and said, "oh, I never add tomatoes to my stew." Then, in a flurry of chopping, talking, and cooking, we were off to the races. Family dinners are a requirement at the parents' house, and naturally we talked about food. Dad's a hot spice junkie, and he proceeded to tell us how adding heat to this dish is particularly important to help your immune system. We looked at each other, pleased that our inner circle gets us! We'd been staring at our computer screens all day and our Qi was more than depleted. This recipe hit all the marks, and it was so good we had seconds, and then ate it for breakfast the next day.

Topping tip: Top with a pinch of cayenne pepper as an added Qi and immunity booster.

Serves 4

- » 3-4 tbsp tapioca flour
- » ¼ tsp each salt and freshly ground black pepper
- » 1 lb organic stewing beef
- » 1-2 tbsp olive oil
- » 1 large onion, diced
- » 2 stalks organic celery, chopped
- » 2 tbsp balsamic vinegar
- » 4 large carrots, chopped into ½-inch pieces
- » 3 cups organic baby potatoes

- » 2 bay leaves
- » ½ tsp thyme
- » ½ tsp dried rosemary (or 1 sprig fresh)
- » 1 tsp Worcestershire sauce (gluten-free, if possible)
- » 3-4 cups organic beef or vegetable broth
- » 1 cup fresh or frozen peas
- » salt and freshly ground black pepper, to taste
- » pinch chili powder, for serving (optional)

Stove-top version

1. In a large bowl, whisk together the tapioca flour, salt, and pepper. Toss in the beef, to coat.
2. In a large (8-quart) stock pot, heat half the oil over medium heat and fry half the beef for about 10 minutes, stirring occasionally, until browned. Transfer the first batch to a bowl using a slotted spoon, and add a splash more oil to the pot to brown the next batch. Transfer the second batch to the bowl.
3. In the same pot over medium heat, sauté the onion and celery, stirring occasionally, for about 5 minutes, until softened. Pour in the vinegar and cook for another 2 minutes, stirring and scraping up the browned bits.
4. Return the beef mixture and any accumulated juices to the pot. Add the carrots, potatoes, bay leaves, thyme, rosemary, Worcestershire sauce, and broth. Bring to a boil, stirring and scraping to loosen any remaining browned bits. Reduce the heat to minimum, cover, and simmer for 3 to 4 hours, stirring occasionally and checking that it's not burning.

5. During the last hour, take the lid off to help reduce the liquid and thicken the stew. At the end, pour in the peas, stir, and serve.

Slow-cooker version

1. In a small bowl, whisk together the tapioca flour with a small amount of broth until well combined.
2. Place all ingredients in the slow cooker, except the peas. Pour in the tapioca mixture and stir to combine. Cover and cook on high for 4 hours or low for 8 hours.
3. When the meat is falling apart, it's ready. Add the peas, stir, and serve.

Qi-Building Desserts

Vanilla Strawberry Apple Crisp

Let's face it, when you're Qi Deficient, you crave sweets. Well, you can eat your fill of this sweet, satisfying, classic crisp. And don't just save it for dessert; it's equally delicious for breakfast. Go on, we dare you to mix it up! This is YOUR journey to (re)awakening your body's healing powers.

Serves 4

Fruit
- » 3-4 organic apples, cored and chopped
- » 2 cups strawberries
- » ½ cup coconut palm (or organic) sugar
- » 3 tbsp tapioca flour

Crumble
- » 1½ cups organic rolled oats
- » ½ cup brown rice flour
- » 3 tbsp maple (or brown rice) syrup
- » ½ cup organic butter, melted
- » 1 tsp pure vanilla extract

1. Preheat the oven to 350°F.
2. For the fruit filling, in a medium bowl toss together the apples, strawberries, half of the sugar (¼ cup), and the tapioca flour. Spread the mixture into an 8 by 8-inch glass or ceramic baking dish.

3. For the crumble, in a medium bowl, combine the oats, brown rice flour, and the remaining ¼ cup of sugar. Pour in the maple syrup, melted butter, and vanilla, and mix until evenly distributed.
4. Sprinkle the crumble mixture over the fruit in the baking dish. Bake for 50 to 60 minutes, or until the top is golden brown and the fruit mixture is bubbling.

Orange Cranberry Scones

A hot cup of tea and the sweet smell of scones baking in the oven, this is what dreams are made of! Especially if your dream is to feel energized and at ease in your body, with a robust and healthy immune system. Zesty and all things scrumptious, these scones are not only a luscious dessert. You can also pack them in your lunch for an afternoon pick-me-up.

Makes 8 scones

- 1½ cups quick-cooking rolled oats, ground fine in blender or coffee grinder
- ½ cup brown rice flour
- ½ tapioca flour
- ¼ cup coconut palm (or organic) sugar
- 1 tbsp baking powder
- zest of one organic orange
- ½ cup organic butter, frozen for at least two hours
- ½ cup dried cranberries
- ¼ cup quick-cooking rolled oats
- 1 organic egg
- ½ cup almond (or coconut) milk
- coconut cream (or whipped coconut cream) for serving (optional)

1. Preheat the oven to 425°F. Have a parchment-paper lined baking sheet on hand.
2. In a medium bowl, combine the ground oats, brown rice flour, tapioca flour, sugar, baking powder, and orange zest.
3. Grate the frozen butter with the largest grooves on your grater. Combine with the flour mixture until coarse and crumbly.
4. Stir in the cranberries and the ¼ cup rolled oats.
5. In a small bowl, beat the egg. Whisk in the milk and pour into the flour mixture, stirring gently until combined, being sure not to over mix. The less you handle the batter, the more melt-in-your-mouth it'll be.
6. Dust a clean work surface with brown rice flour and press the dough out into a 1-inch-thick circle. Cut it into 8 even pizza-shaped wedges.
7. Place the wedges on the baking sheet and bake for 15 minutes, until the scones are beginning to turn golden brown. They'll be very delicate and crumbly fresh out of the oven, so let them cool on a rack a bit before eating.
8. To make this out-of-this-world delicious, serve with coconut cream, especially when hot out of the oven.

Qi Stagnation Reset

What's Happening in Your Body when You Have Qi Stagnation?

You might feel like you're stuck in that proverbial rut, spinning your wheels and watching life pass you by.

We're here to tell you that this rut is not proverbial at all. Qi Stagnation is very real, and the sense of being stuck is only slightly more pleasant than banging your head against a wall.

Maybe you've landed here feeling stuck in work, love, or money and you're tired of life happening around you. Maybe you feel like no matter how hard you try, it's hard for you to move forward.

Picture this: you have another great new idea at work. You run it by a few of your colleagues, as you always do, and you feel like "this is it," you're going to make your career mark.

You present the idea to your boss, and they put up their hand, interrupting you mid-sentence: "We'll have to think about it, maybe next time." Now you're pissed, but somehow the anger doesn't move you forward. Though you're starting to question your career, fear pulls you back into inertia.

Now, imagine 10 years go by. You're still at the same company, and nothing has changed because you're afraid to stick your neck out. You clock in and out for a paycheque and wonder "Is this as good as it gets?"

Cheer up, kiddo, you just have Qi Stagnation. The good news is it's MOVABLE! We're gonna get you UNstuck.

In Traditional Chinese Medicine, Qi Stagnation is a constriction or suppression of emotional and creative energy. We stifle our sense of self and try to be who we think others want us to be. This may start with early trauma, but eventually it becomes a self-generating pattern. In other words, holding stuff in gets you – and your Qi – stuck.

Qi (say chee) drives movement and fluidity in the body, so stuck or stagnant Qi leads to a cascade of events. Once we've suppressed our feelings for long enough, physical symptoms begin to appear. Unfortunately, we often seek help only after symptoms start to manifest in our bodies.

Physically, you might experience pain, irritable bowel syndrome (IBS), hormonal imbalance, or a lump in your throat.

Emotionally, Qi Stagnation can cause you to feel frustrated, irritable, depressed, and/or anxious. A lifetime of not expressing your emotions and creativity is what gets you feeling stuck. Whatever your physical and emotional symptoms, the root of Qi Stagnation is in holding back your creativity – suppressing the RAW expression of who you truly are. Initially, this is probably imposed on you by family, society, or some "authority," but once you've internalized it to the point that your sense of ALIVENESS is chronically suppressed, Qi Stagnation sets in.

What Qi Stagnation can look like

Candice is a classic Type A personality, an overachieving perfectionist who thrives on running a tight, efficient ship and piling lots on her plate. At least, she *thinks* she's thriving. Really, all is not well.

Here are the signs that Candice needs the Qi Stagnation Reset:

- High anxiety, stressed out
- Mood swings, including easily irritated and angry
- Borderline depression in spite of being on antidepressants
- Extreme PMS, sometimes two weeks out of the month
- Irregular stop-start periods with lots of spotting
- Tender breasts (a Stagnation giveaway)
- Headaches
- Wakes between 1 and 3 a.m. with busy mind and can't get back to sleep
- Constipation, lack of hunger

Candice looks slim and healthy, but she's skipping meals and running on coffee and Coke. She gets quickly exhausted, but somehow she can always power through. On the outside she looks like our culture's ideal high achiever. She always gets the job done. But on the inside she is catastrophizing, controlling, and uptight, and she has no idea how to relax.

Here's how Candice will know the Qi Stagnation Reset is working:

- More relaxed and at ease, but still in control
- Periods more consistent, no breast tenderness
- More stable mood
- Fewer headaches
- Better sleep
- More able to slow down and nourish herself

Goals for Moving Qi

Resolving Qi Stagnation and breaking out of old patterns can feel risky. Let's face it, change on any level is hard.

Here's the easy part: getting your Qi moving again depends on FUN. The key to shifting stagnation is to follow your interests, hobbies, and passions.

What if, instead of looking at life through the rearview mirror, you could rekindle the childlike wonder that's deep inside you? Remember those dusty old tap shoes you've kept all these years because they remind you of the happiest days of your life? Well, bust 'em out and get tapping. This is the true essence of finding your inner child. Go back to the time and place you were FREE to be YOU. This is the key to unlocking the inner prison you're living in and busting out.

Breaking up Qi Stagnation means letting things roll off your back in an imperfectly human kind of way. And a little note for parents: maybe your kids don't need you to be perfect. Maybe they just want you to show up and be happy.

Kitchen Medicine for Moving Qi

Give yourself a pat on the back for showing up here. We're going to get you eating the foods that will restore your gut-brain connection, increase your body's energy, and rebalance your mind and emotions.

Essentially, to free up your Qi with food, we want you to lighten up. Here are your key words for foods that alleviate Qi Stagnation:

- Young and tender veggies
- Sour
- Fermented

Think of springtime veggies like asparagus, chives, and tender young salad greens. Raw living sprouted and fermented foods are perfect for moving your Qi. Think sourdough bread made from wild yeasts, or kombucha and sauerkraut.

When it comes to fruit, we want you to go light and sour, like grapefruit, rhubarb, and apricots. The lightness is easy to digest and the sour taste is great for breaking up symptoms of stagnation like PMS, irritability, and depression.

The idea is to avoid foods that are heavy, rich, and high in fat: fatty meats, cream, cheese, eggs, and an excess of nuts and seeds.

How do you feel after eating these heavy foods? Probably kind of heavy, right? We could also call this sluggish and stagnant. These foods definitely have a place in your diet, but if you're experiencing symptoms of Qi Stagnation, they're not your friends right now. By removing them just for now (this is a reset, not a lifetime diet), you can clear the sludge and get things flowing freely again.

As you begin tasting and experimenting with the recipes, you'll get the hang of what unsticks you. You'll notice how buoyant and healthy you feel when you eat green foods, especially bitter greens. And did you get the memo about sour and bitter foods being good for stimulating your liver and digestion? Imagine bitters helping to break down your food and break up that stagnant energy in your body.

So, there you have it, the foods that'll help you lighten up and get your Qi moving again so you can step into the full expression of your most gorgeous, juicy self.

Getting Started with Moving Qi

You're here because you've identified Qi Stagnation as your main imbalance. You can also turn to this diet during early spring or any time you want to get back on track after an overindulgence (hello, winter-holiday food hangovers!).

Foods in the Qi Stagnation diet are light, fresh, and delicious. Your brain responds to the deep, rich colours of young shoots and greens and lightly cooked, tangy flavours from around the world! We can even promise a revolutionary new take on that childhood favourite, chicken noodle soup (see Glass Noodle Soup with Herb-Spiced Meatballs, page 268).

Activities for Moving Qi

With Qi Stagnation, you need to get things moving. Exercise is essential for your physical and emotional body. Moving three times a week is ideal, but make it movement you LOVE.

Your many great options include:

- Walking with a friend (or dreaming while you walk)
- Hiking in nature
- High-intensity interval training (HIIT)
- Yoga, especially vinyasa, kundalini, and hatha
- Dancing – pick up some new moves on YouTube!
- Swimming
- Any sports

Which ones get you a little excited? Start with those.

Another great way to get your Qi moving is to exercise your creativity. Did you let go of a hobby you loved because you got too busy? Is there something you've always dreamed of trying? This is your time to pick up a journal or some knitting needles, start an indoor sprout garden, or dig out those paints. But whatever you choose, do it with a childlike spirit. This is NOT about getting it "right" or being productive.

In other words, we are prescribing FUN as one of the key medicines for releasing those feelings of being stuck. Take yourself out on what Julia Cameron, author of *The*

Artist's Way, calls an "artist's date": buy yourself some new art supplies or browse a craft fair or art gallery. Watch comedy and laugh!

Beverages that Move Qi

So many tasty ways to drink your Qi into action! Sour, naturally fermented beverages have to be at the top of the list. Naturally fermented kombucha and water kefir are wonderful options for drinking your medicine. Mint is also great for stagnation, as are lemon and lime. So, go ahead and fill up a pitcher of water, toss in fresh mint leaves, and add a few squeezes of lemon or lime, then sip throughout the day.

Daily green drink – One glass wheatgrass (or spirulina/chlorella) following serving size on the bottle.

Herbal coffee – Dandy Blend (we love this coffee substitute)

Kombucha – This delightful bubbly fermented drink is fun to drink and delicious. Enjoy daily or on special occasions.

Herbal and medicinal teas – See "How to make medicinal teas" on page 61. Look for these herbs and blends from Traditional Medicinals:

- Mint
- Linden with Hawthorne & Lemon Balm
- Chamomile and Lavender
- Dandelion Leaf and Root
- Green Tea

Also try Organic India Tulsi Teas Tulsi Rose (Holy Basil).

Qi Stagnation Reset Food Chart

Fruits	Vegetables	More Vegetables
Apricots	Arugula	Sprouts
Grapefruit	Asparagus	Taro root
Lemons	Beets	Turnips
Limes	Broccoli	Watercress
Organic cherries	Cabbage	
Organic grapes	Carrots	
Organic green apples	Cucumbers	
	Fennel	**Grains**
Organic peaches	Garlic	
Organic strawberries	Green onions	Amaranth
Plums	Kelp	Millet
Raspberries	Kohlrabi	Quinoa
Rhubarb	Leafy greens	Rice
	Lettuce	Rye
	Mushrooms	Sourdough
	Onions	Sprouted grains
	Organic celery	Sweet rice
	Radish/Daikon	

Digestion tips: Incorporate a herbal bitter before each meal. Salus Gallexier Herbal Bitters and St. Francis Canadian Bitters are good. Even having a couple pieces of grapefruit will help to stimulate di-

Organic Protein	Additional	Foods to Avoid
Chicken	Apple cider vinegar	Eggs
Edamame	Kombucha	GMO foods
Fish	Licorice root	Non organic foods
Flax seeds	Pickles in brine	Processed foods
Legumes	Raw honey	Red meat
Mung beans	Sauerkraut	Spicy foods
Pine nuts	Stevia	Alcohol
Pulses		Animal fats
Pumpkin seeds	**Herbs**	Buckwheat
Soy*		Coffee
Sunflower seeds	Basil	Dairy
Tempeh	Bay leaf	
Tofu	Chives	
	Cilantro	
	Dill	
	Marjoram	
* Ideally	Mint	
Sprouted pulses and legumes	Rosemary	

gestion. Finish your meal with either a pickle in brine (not the ones in vinegar), a small scoop of sauerkraut, or a cup of tea (see page 61).

Sample Qi-Moving Meal Plans

Day 1

Breakfast: Raspberry Peach Smoothie and a cup of green tea
Snack: Lemon Lime Strawberry Muffins
Lunch: Dill Tuna Salad with Lemon Avocado Mayo
Snack: Trail mix: pumpkin seeds, pine nuts, sunflower seeds with dried plums and peaches
Dinner: Roasted Squash & Quinoa Bowls with Tangy Nut Sauce

Day 2

Breakfast: Roasted Squash & Quinoa Bowls with Tangy Nut Sauce
Snack: Strawberry Jam and pumpkin seed butter rice cake sandwich
Lunch: Smoked Fakin' Bacon Club Sandwich
Snack: Organic kale chips
Dinner: Glass Noodle Soup with Herb-Spiced Meatballs

More Snack Options

- Fresh fruit breakfast bowl and cup of green tea
- Apricot Banana Breakfast Cookies and serving of wheatgrass drink
- Cashew Coconut Crusted Lime Tart
- Grapefruit sprinkled with raw cane sugar

Day 3

Breakfast: Fresh Dill & Mushroom Tofu Scramble
Snack: Rice crackers and pumpkin seed butter and cup of Dandy Blend coffee substitute
Lunch: White Bean Cucumber & Tomato Salad
Snack: Popcorn sprinkled with spirulina powder and nutritional yeast
Dinner: Lemon Lime Roast Chicken

Day 4

Breakfast: Raspberry Peach Smoothie
Snack: Apricot Banana Breakfast Cookies and cup of tea: Linden with Hawthorn and Lemon Balm tea
Lunch: Lemony Cucumber Raw Kale Salad
Snack: Green apple slices and sunflower seed butter
Dinner: Hawaiian Tofu Poké with Fresh Greens

More Snack Options

- Trail mix: pumpkin seeds, pine nuts, sunflower seeds with dried apples and strawberries
- Organic kale chips and glass of kombucha
- Cup of miso soup with tofu
- Vanilla Bean Chia Pudding

Qi Stagnation Breakfasts

Apricot Banana Breakfast Cookies

Want your family to love you more? Let them eat cookies for breakfast! Or, better yet, teach them to make these cookies to make your mornings easier. And be sure to make them big and hearty, 'cause mama needs to eat. This is breakfast after all — one of our three favourite meals.

Preparation tip: Make sure the batter is wet, but not too runny.

Protein tip: To boost your protein, pair with our Raspberry Peach Smoothie on page 241.

Makes 1 dozen

- » 2 very ripe bananas, mashed (riper = better flavour)
- » 2 tbsp almond (or sunflower seed) butter
- » ½–1 tbsp raw honey
- » 1 cup gluten-free rolled oats
- » ½ cup dried apricots, chopped into small pieces (or dried organic strawberries, peaches, plums, or cherries)

1. Preheat the oven to 350°F. Grease a baking sheet with butter, coconut oil, or olive oil, or line with parchment paper.
2. In a medium bowl, mash the bananas with a fork or potato masher until almost smooth (some lumps are okay). Stir in the almond butter and honey until well combined.

3. Pour in the rolled oats and mix. Then toss in the dried apricots and stir until combined.
4. Spoon onto the prepared baking sheet and bake for 15 to 20 minutes. They'll still be soft and won't really brown, so just bake until they firm up. Let cool on a rack before eating.

Raspberry Peach Smoothie

If you wake up feeling a bit sluggish on Day 2 or 3, this light, refreshing smoothie will balance your blood sugar, unburden your liver, and get your Qi flowing freely again. You'll be bursting with energy and ready to take on your day. (Flip over to page 49 to get all the deets on how we use smoothies to heal.)

Ingredient tip: Using fresh raspberries and peaches is ideal in this recipe. If you do use frozen fruit, pull it out of the freezer and let it thaw a little. (To speed up the process, you can put the sealed bag or container in a warm-water bath.) Warming the fruit will help you absorb the sweet and tart energetic properties of this drink more easily.

Serves 1

- ½ green-tipped banana, cut into pieces (optional)
- ½ cup raspberries
- 1 peach
- 1 cup almond milk
- 1-2 cup water
- 1 scoop protein powder (see page 48 for options)
- 1 tbsp ground flax seeds (optional)

1. Place all the ingredients into a blender or Vitamix and blend for a good 30 seconds, or until velvety smooth.

Fresh Dill & Mushroom Tofu Scramble

We know what you're thinking, "meh, tofu scramble." But this light, fluffy dish is seriously delicious and, thanks to the turmeric, it even looks like scrambled eggs. The fresh dill not only makes the flavour of this dish, it's highly therapeutic.

Ingredient tip: Get more from your scramble by using coarse-grained Dijon mustard made with apple cider vinegar. Vinegar is amazing at breaking up Qi Stagnation.
Serving tip: Go all out and dish this up with roasted fingerling potatoes and asparagus.

Serves 4

- 2 tbsp olive oil
- 1 small onion, diced
- 1 cup thinly sliced mushrooms (button or your choice)
- 1 tbsp organic tamari soy sauce (or Bragg Liquid Aminos)
- 1 tbsp grainy mustard
- 1 tbsp water
- ½ tsp ground turmeric
- 1 lb organic extra-firm tofu, pressed dry and crumbled
- ½ cup organic cherry tomatoes, sliced in half
- ½ cup minced fresh dill

1. In a large frying pan, heat the olive oil over medium heat. Sauté the onion and mushrooms for 3 to 5 minutes, until the onion is translucent.
2. In a medium bowl, combine the soy sauce, mustard, water, and turmeric. Toss in the crumbled tofu and combine well.
3. Pour the tofu mixture into the pan and cook for about 5 minutes, stirring occasionally. Take off the heat and stir in the tomatoes and fresh dill.

Lemon Lime Strawberry Muffins

Vegan muffins? Fear not, friends, this recipe will be a keeper. The hardest part of transitioning to healthful eating is getting started. We promise that once your pantry is fully stocked with these nutrient-dense flours, you'll be searching for other recipes that use them.

Ingredient tip: Use whatever fruit you have on hand as long as it's in the Qi Stagnation food chart (page 232).
Protein Tip: To boost your protein, pair with our Raspberry Peach Smoothie on page 241.

Makes 1 dozen

Dry
- » 1½ cups brown rice flour
- » ½ cup tapioca flour
- » 2 tsp baking powder
- » ½ tsp baking soda

Wet
- » 2 bananas, mashed
- » ½ cup coconut palm (or organic) sugar
- » ¼ cup melted organic virgin coconut (or avocado) oil
- » 1 cup almond (or soy) milk
- » 2 tbsp chia seeds, ground in a coffee grinder or Vitamix
- » zest of one lemon (top layer only, not bitter white underneath)
- » zest of ½ lime (top layer)

» ¾ cup diced strawberries

1. Preheat the oven to 350°F. Grease a 12-cup muffin tin, or do as we do and line with paper cups.
2. Combine the dry ingredients in a medium bowl.
3. In a second medium bowl, whisk together the bananas, sugar, oil, milk, ground chia, and zests. Let the mixture sit for a few minutes to thicken up, then stir again.
4. Slowly add the dry ingredients into the wet and stir until combined. Fold in the strawberries.
5. Pour the batter into the prepared tin and bake for 35 minutes, or until a knife inserted in the centre comes out almost clean (they'll still be a bit moist). Cool and enjoy.

Qi Stagnation Lunches

Smoked Fakin' Bacon Club Sandwich

Looking for a vegan BLT? Look no further. Tempeh is an acquired taste, but you'll be able to trick all the bacon lovers in your family with this sammie. Trust us, they'll be hooked.

Ingredient tips: For extra deliciousness, be sure to really brown your tempeh to give it a good crunch. If you want fewer carbs or a lighter meal, go for a lettuce leaf wrap instead of bread.

Serves 3

- » 1 package organic smoked tempeh (called "smoked" or "bacon flavoured")
- » 1 tsp olive oil
- » sliced rye sourdough (or gluten-free) bread
- » honey mustard (or add a little honey to Dijon or grainy mustard)
- » 1 organic tomato, sliced
- » 1 avocado, sliced lengthwise
- » 1 package organic alfalfa or other sprouts (or watercress)
- » sea salt and freshly ground black pepper, to taste

1. Slice the tempeh into ⅛-inch slices, the thinner the better for the crisping-up factor.

2. In a medium frying pan, heat the oil over medium heat and fry the tempeh slices for about 1 to 3 minutes on each side, until golden brown.
3. Toast the bread, spread with the mustard, and top with the tomato, avocado, sprouts, and cooked tempeh. Seriously yum!

Dill Tuna Salad with Lemon Avocado Mayo

This modern twist on a classic sandwich is delicious, creamy, and crunchy. Chock full of omega oils (good fats) and fresh dill (the best herb in your grocery store), this is guaranteed to lift you out of that Qi-Stagnation rut.

Serving tip: Add a pickle in brine (not vinegar) on the side to double the healing properties and boost your digestion.

Serves 2

Tuna salad
- » 1 can tuna, drained and flaked (we use Raincoat Trading brand)
- » ½–1 avocado, mashed
- » 1 small stalk organic celery, finely diced (about ¼ cup)
- » 2 tbsp finely diced red onion
- » 1 tbsp minced fresh dill (1 tsp dried)
- » juice of ½ lemon
- » pinch of sea salt
- » freshly ground black pepper

For serving
- » rye, sourdough, or gluten-free bread slices, toasted
- » tomato slices
- » alfalfa sprouts
- » Dijon or grainy mustard (optional)

1. In a medium bowl, combine the tuna and mashed avocado and mix well. Add the celery, red onion, dill, and lemon juice, and season with salt and pepper.
2. Scoop onto toasted bread and top with tomato slices, sprouts, and a little mustard, if you'd like. Crunchalicious!

Lemony Cucumber Raw Kale Salad

The secret to a yummy raw kale salad is massaging the leaves with olive oil. This softens the kale so it can be digested more easily and infused with other flavours. We also recommend choosing bunches that are crisp, young, and tender. This healing salad stays bright and delicious for days, and you'll have leftover dressing!

Ingredient tip: If you're planning to eat this over the week, hold the avocado and add it just before serving.
Protein tip: Serve with fresh grilled meat or fish or some pan-fried tempeh to meet your protein needs.

Serves 4

- » 4 cups cooked quinoa (1½ cups uncooked)

Salad
- » 1 bunch organic kale
- » 1 tbsp olive oil
- » ½ cucumber, thinly sliced
- » 4-6 radishes, thinly sliced
- » 1 avocado, diced into small cubes

Dressing
- » juice of 1 lemon
- » ⅓ cup olive oil
- » 1 clove garlic, minced
- » ½ tsp Dijon mustard
- » 2 tsp maple syrup (or honey)
- » pinch of sea salt and freshly ground black pepper

1. Cook the quinoa according to package directions.
2. For the salad, wash and dry the kale. Pull the leaves from the thick stems and tear into bite-sized pieces. Heap the kale in a large bowl, drizzle with 1 tbsp oil, and massage with your hands. The leaves will begin to shrink and turn dark emerald green. Toss in the cucumber, radishes, and avocado.
3. For the dressing, in a small mixing bowl whisk together all the ingredients until well combined.
4. Pour half the dressing (or to taste) over the salad, and serve over a bed of cooked quinoa.

White Bean Cucumber & Tomato Salad

This simple, light salad will keep you coming back for more. An easy, stand-alone, refreshing meal or a side to your main dish, this salad looks gorgeous and tastes delicious. Oh, and it moves your Qi. Win, win, win!

Serving tip: Serve at your next party as a dip. Call it a "chunky bean salsa," and grab a bag of organic blue corn tortilla chips for scooping it up.

Serves 3-4

- 2 14-oz cans organic navy beans (or any small white bean)
- 1 small cucumber, diced
- 1 large organic tomato, diced
- 1 organic yellow bell pepper, diced
- ½ cup minced parsley
- 3 tbsp olive oil
- 1 tbsp organic tamari soy sauce (or Bragg Liquid Aminos)
- juice of ½-1 lemon
- ½ tbsp maple syrup
- sea salt and freshly ground black pepper, to taste

1. In a medium bowl, toss together the beans, cucumber, tomato, pepper, and parsley. Drizzle oil on top and mix.
2. Add the soy sauce, ½ the lemon juice, and the maple syrup. Toss to combine. Season with salt, pepper, and a little more lemon juice, to taste.
3. Great to eat right away, but it really soaks up the flavours if you let it sit for a couple of hours.

Qi Stagnation Dinners

Lemon Lime Roast Chicken

Keep this recipe in your back pocket for dinner parties. Tangy and fresh, with a nice sticky sweetness, this healthy twist on honey garlic chicken will wow your guests. Go ahead and double the recipe, you'll want leftovers for tomorrow's lunch. Along with the flavour kick comes serious health benefits, as lemons and limes are probably the best fruits for detoxifying you from overconsumption (hello, holiday parties and winter overeating). Serve this up with pan-roasted asparagus and a fluffy mound of quinoa or mashed dill potatoes.

Ingredient tip: You can substitute a whole butterflied chicken for the thighs.

Serves 6

- » zest and juice of 1 lemon
- » zest and juice of 1 lime
- » 3 cloves garlic, minced
- » 1 tbsp minced ginger root
- » ¼ cup raw honey
- » ¼ cup olive oil
- » ½ tsp sea salt
- » freshly ground black pepper
- » 6 organic chicken thighs, bone in, skin on

1. Preheat the oven to 375°F.
2. In a large bowl, combine all the ingredients except the chicken.

3. Add the chicken and toss to coat. Cover and marinate in the fridge for at least 30 minutes, ideally up to 8 hours.
4. Place the marinated chicken thighs in a large casserole dish, skin-side up. Bake, uncovered, for 30 to 40 minutes, or until the thighs are well browned and cooked through.

Roasted Squash & Quinoa Bowls with Tangy Nut Sauce

This is the ultimate dish to help counteract overindulgence. (Yes, we all do it.) Delicata squash may be hard to find, but it's what helps create the lightness and easy-to-digest factors we need after a night, or more, of excess consumption.

Zucchini tip: Zucchini is one of the top GMO foods so we strongly recommend buying organic. Your liver and hormones will thank you.

Serves 4

Squash & filling
- » 3 delicata squash, roasted (acorn and butternut work well too)
- » 1 cup quinoa (3 cups cooked)
- » 2 medium organic zucchini

Tangy nut sauce
- » ½ cup nut butter (almond, sunflower seed, cashew)
- » ½ cup water
- » 1 tbsp organic tamari soy sauce (or Bragg Liquid Aminos)
- » 1 tbsp apple cider vinegar
- » ½ tbsp sesame oil
- » ½ tbsp maple syrup (or honey)
- » 1 clove garlic, minced

1. Preheat the oven to 425°F.
2. Roast the whole squashes until they are soft and fork tender, about 45 minutes. Slice them lengthwise and scoop out the seeds.
3. Meanwhile, cook the quinoa according to package directions, or rinse well and cook in twice as much water. Grate the zucchini.
4. To make the sauce, in a small bowl whisk together all the tangy nut sauce ingredients.
5. To assemble, scoop the cooked quinoa into the hollowed part of each squash. Top with the raw zucchini, drizzle with the sauce, and serve.

Carrot Dill Soup

This soup does not discriminate: it's a crowd pleaser for both vegans and meat eaters. The potatoes make it hearty, but you could also add a scoop of any cooked grain from the food chart (page 232). Don't skip the fresh dill. It's highly therapeutic and makes the soup taste delicious.

Serves 4

- » 2 tbsp olive oil
- » 1 small onion, chopped
- » 3 stalks organic celery, chopped (about 1 cup)
- » 10–12 carrots, chopped (about 6 cups)
- » 2 small organic Yukon gold potatoes, chopped
- » 6 cups organic chicken or vegetable broth
- » ½ cup minced fresh dill
- » sea salt and freshly ground black pepper, to taste

1. In a large saucepan, heat the olive oil over medium heat and sauté the onion for 1 to 2 minutes, until translucent. Add the celery, carrots, and potatoes, and cook for another 5 minutes, stirring occasionally.
2. Add the broth and bring to a boil. Reduce the heat, cover the pot, and simmer for about 25 minutes, or until the vegetables are tender.
3. Remove from the heat and blend until smooth using either an immersion blender or Vitamix.
4. Stir in the fresh dill and season with salt and pepper, if necessary.

Fish Tacos with Pickled Red Onions & Avocado Salsa

It's the end of the week and you're dying to get the weekend started. This light, refreshing recipe will have you singing "La Bamba" as you assemble your taco and reach for your wine glass of kombucha. After 30 minutes of prep, all you need is 10 minutes to cook and steam the tortillas, and mere seconds to assemble and chow down.

Pickled onion tip: Prepare the pickled onions a minimum of 2 hours in advance, or even the day before. Once you taste these tangy morsels, you'll be adding them to sandwiches, salads, and anything else you can think of.

Serves 4

Pickled onions
- ½ cup olive oil
- 1-2 tbsp apple cider vinegar
- 1 small red onion, finely sliced
- freshly ground black pepper

Fish
- 1 lb firm wild white fish fillets
- juice of ½ lime
- 2 tbsp olive oil, plus 1 tbsp for frying
- 1 clove garlic, minced
- sea salt and freshly ground black pepper

Salsa
- 1 avocado, diced
- 2 tbsp finely diced organic sweet bell pepper

- » 2 tbsp finely diced red onion
- » juice of ½ lime
- » sea salt and freshly ground black pepper

For serving
- » organic soft corn or gluten-free tortillas (fresh or frozen)
- » 1 pint organic alfalfa sprouts

1. At least 2 hours before serving, prepare the pickled onions. In a small bowl, whisk together the oil and vinegar and toss in the onion slices. Season with pepper and cover with plastic wrap. Set aside for the onions to mellow out and become translucent red.
2. Meanwhile, prepare the fish. Place the fillets in a shallow dish (like a pie plate) and squeeze the lime juice over them. Sprinkle with 2 tablespoons of the oil and the garlic, salt, and pepper, and marinate in the fridge for about 20 minutes.
3. Preheat the oven to 400°F.
4. In a large frying pan, heat the remaining 1 tablespoon of olive oil over medium heat. Cook the fish for about 3 minutes on each side, or until done. Remove from the pan and set aside.
5. To prepare the salsa, in a small bowl combine all the ingredients, mixing well.
6. Remove the onions from the dressing. You can use the dressing to drizzle on the tacos, if you like.
7. Heat the tortillas in the oven for 1 to 2 minutes, until warm but still soft.
8. To serve, spoon some fish onto each tortilla and top with the salsa, onions, and sprouts.

Fresh Green Salsa & Mexican Tostadas

This TCM twist on the Mexican classic is propelled into an instant favourite by the crunchy tortillas with spiced beans and fresh-herbed salsa. The green salsa also livens up fish and rice dishes.

Tortilla tip: If you can find blue corn tortillas, get 'em. From the TCM perspective, their greater cooling effect and slightly sour taste make them more effective than yellow corn at moving your Qi. Blue corn is a win according to western nutrition too. It contains 21 percent more protein, 50 percent more iron, and 2 times the manganese and potassium of yellow corn. The best thing about blue corn is that it's never been a GMO crop, so it's still in its pure form, like the grain our ancestors ate.

Serves 4

Salsa
- 1 small onion, chopped
- 1 bunch cilantro, chopped
- 1 small jalapeno, deseeded and chopped (omit if you're feeding children or don't like heat)
- 2 cloves garlic, chopped
- 1 small organic yellow pepper, chopped
- ¼ cup olive oil
- 2 tbsp apple cider vinegar
- 2 tsp oregano
- 1 tsp ground coriander
- ½ tsp sea salt
- freshly ground black pepper

Filling
- ¼ cup water
- 1 19-oz can adzuki (or kidney or pinto) beans (2 cups cooked)
- 2 tsp chili powder (or ½ tsp each paprika, oregano, cumin, and garlic powder, with pinch of cayenne pepper)
- pinch sea salt

To serve
- organic soft corn or gluten-free tortillas (fresh or frozen)
- olive oil, for brushing tortillas
- 1 organic tomato, diced
- 1 avocado, diced
- watercress (or any sprouts)

1. Preheat the oven to 400°F.
2. To prepare the salsa, combine all ingredients in a blender or Vitamix. Blend to a pesto-like smoothness.
3. In a small frying pan, combine the water, beans, and chili powder over medium heat. Simmer for about 5 minutes, stirring regularly. Take off the heat and mash into a paste with a potato masher (a bit chunky is fine).
4. Brush the tortillas with olive oil and place on a baking sheet. Heat for about 3 to 5 minutes on each side until crispy.
5. To serve, spread some beans onto each tortilla and top with a scoop of green salsa, avocado, tomato, and watercress or sprouts.

Glass Noodle Soup with Herb-Spiced Meatballs

"So long" classic chicken noodle soup and "Hello" food-formula glass noodle soup. This is the new-and-improved version of chicken soup for the soul. Eating a bowl will warm you up and nourish every cell in your body. You'll want to keep it all to yourself, but we encourage you to share it with family and friends.

Substitution tip: Use ½ cup leftover grain, either quinoa or rice, as a substitute for the puffed rice cereal.

Noodle tip: Look for Longkou Vermicelli, a common brand of mung bean vermicelli (cellophane noodles) found in the international section of most grocery stores.

Serves 4

Meatballs
- 1 lb ground organic turkey
- 1 garlic clove, minced
- 3 green onions, finely chopped
- 1 tsp dried basil
- ½ tsp dried oregano
- ½ tsp sea salt
- freshly ground black pepper
- ½ cup puffed rice cereal, ground in food processor/coffee grinder (or any gluten-free flour)
- 2 tbsp olive oil

Soup
- » 8 cups organic chicken (or vegetable) broth
- » 2 carrots, sliced
- » 2 stalks organic celery, sliced
- » 3 bunches mung bean vermicelli (cellophane noodles)
- » 3 cups organic kale, chopped

1. In a medium bowl, combine the ground turkey, garlic, green onions, basil, oregano, salt, pepper, and ground rice cereal. Roll into about 16 1-inch meatballs.
2. In a large frying pan, heat the olive oil over medium heat and brown the meatballs on all sides. Remove from the pan and drain on a paper-towel-lined plate.
3. In a large pot, bring the broth to a boil. Add the browned meatballs, reduce the heat, and simmer for 10 minutes.
4. Add the carrots, celery, and vermicelli and cook for another 4 minutes, or until the noodles are cooked. Stir in the kale, turn off the heat, and serve immediately!

Thai Fried Rice with Fresh Herbs

Cook your way around the globe without leaving your kitchen. This plant-based dish features whole foods and exotic flavours, and we're warning you: it just might become your new crave.

Ingredient tips: If you're looking for a variation on the classic Pad Thai, substitute rice noodles for the rice. And do look for fresh mint and basil, because they really make this dish.
Prep tip: Day-old rice is essential, so cook up 2 cups of rice the day before.
Protein tip: Serve with fresh-grilled meat or fish, or some pan-fried tempeh, to meet your protein needs.

Serves 4

Sauce
- » 1–1½ tbsp organic tomato paste
- » 3 tbsp organic tamari soy sauce (or Bragg Liquid Aminos)
- » 2 tbsp sesame oil
- » juice of ½–1 lime
- » zest of one lime (top green layer only, not bitter white underneath)

Rice
- » 1 tbsp olive oil
- » 1 organic yellow bell pepper, chopped
- » 2 cloves garlic, minced
- » 1 tbsp minced ginger root

- » 4 green onions, thinly sliced
- » 6 cups cooked brown rice, prepared the day before
- » 2 tbsp fresh mint
- » 2 tbsp fresh basil
- » ½ cup peeled and finely diced cucumber
- » package of fresh sunflower or pea sprouts

1. To make the sauce, in a small bowl whisk together all ingredients.
2. For the rice, heat the olive oil in a large frying pan over medium heat and sauté the pepper for 3 minutes. Add the garlic and ginger and cook another 2 minutes, stirring frequently. Add the green onions and cook for 30 seconds longer.
3. Break the day-old rice into medium-sized clumps and toss into the pan. Pour the sauce over the rice and toss to coat. Stir in the fresh mint and basil and cook for 3 to 5 minutes, or until heated through.
4. Spoon onto plates and top with the cucumber and a handful of sprouts.

Papaya Chicken Avocado Salad with Papaya Seed Vinaigrette

Hello Hawaii, specifically the north shore of Oahu at Uncle Barney's farm in Pupukea. Imagine picking papayas and avocados from the trees and picking up fresh greens and sprouts from the local farmers market. This easy-breezy meal lights up your spirit. A feast for your eyes and taste buds, it's versatile enough to work for lunch or dinner.

Papaya seed tip: Don't throw out those seeds! You can eat them fresh, like in this recipe, or save them by drying or freezing. Fresh seeds have a stronger taste than dried, a little like horseradish or black pepper, spicy and a little bitter. Papaya seeds pack the nutritional punch of antioxidants, fibre, healthy fatty acids, and many health benefits.

Serves 4

Chicken
- 2 boneless organic chicken breasts, skin on
- 1 tbsp olive oil
- sea salt and freshly ground black pepper

Papaya Seed Vinaigrette
- ½ cup olive oil
- 3 tbsp apple cider vinegar
- 2 tbsp papaya seeds
- ¼ cup finely diced white onion
- 2 tbsp honey
- 2 tbsp water

- » ½ tbsp Dijon mustard
- » ¼ tsp sea salt

Salad
- » 8 cups mixed salad greens
- » 1 package sunflower sprouts (pea sprouts are also nice)
- » 1 package organic alfalfa sprouts (or any other sprouts, like garlic or broccoli)
- » 1 avocado, thinly sliced lengthwise
- » 1 organic papaya, cut into 1-inch cubes (save the seeds for the dressing)

1. Preheat the oven to 400°F.
2. Wash the chicken breasts and pat them dry with a paper towel. Drizzle with the olive oil and season with salt and pepper. Place in a glass baking dish and bake for 20 to 25 minutes, or until done. Set aside to cool while you make the salad. Once cool enough to touch, slice or pull the chicken into thin strips.
3. For the vinaigrette, combine all the ingredients in a blender or Vitamix. Blend until smooth, about a minute or two.
4. To assemble, arrange the mixed greens, sprouts, avocado, papaya, and chicken on four plates. Drizzle with the vinaigrette and serve immediately.

Hawaiian Tofu Poké with Fresh Greens

Hawaii, you are forever in our hearts. You inspire us with the plethora of goodies Mother Earth provides wherever the sun shines. Poké is traditionally served with ahi (tuna), but we replaced it with tofu for its Qi-moving benefits. Healing and paradise, all in one bowl!

Ingredient tip: If you have access to fresh ahi tuna, go for it because it's another Qi-mover AND it's delicious!
Prep tip: Make sure you give yourself an extra half hour for the tofu to marinate.

Serves 4

Tofu
- 1 lb extra-firm organic tofu, cut into ½-inch cubes
- 1 tbsp olive oil

Marinade
- ¼ cup organic tamari soy sauce (or Bragg Liquid Aminos)
- 2 tbsp sesame oil
- ⅓ cup diced red onion
- juice of ¼ lemon
- pinch of chili flakes (optional)

For serving
- 6 cups cooked rice
- 4 cups mixed greens
- 2 tbsp sesame seeds
- 1 bunch green onions, finely chopped

1. Pat the tofu dry with paper towels or a clean dish towel. Cut into ½-inch cubes and pat dry again. This is the key to crispy, delicious tofu.
2. In a medium frying pan, heat the oil over medium-high heat. Add the tofu cubes and cook for about 7 to 10 minutes, tossing regularly so they turn a light golden brown on all sides. Set aside on a paper-towel-lined plate to soak up any excess oil.
3. In a medium bowl, combine all the marinade ingredients. Toss in the cooked tofu and refrigerate for at least 30 minutes to marinate.
4. Meanwhile, cook your rice and wash and dry your salad greens.
5. To assemble, toss the green onions and sesame seeds into the marinated tofu and serve over mixed greens, with hot rice on the side. Deeelish!

Qi Stagnation Desserts

Cashew Coconut-Crusted Lime Tart

This is the ultimate pucker-your-lips-with-love dessert. Dazzle your friends with this dish at your next dinner party and watch as joy lights up their faces. You may even get them curious about Yin Yang Reset with this palate cleanser and Qi mover. Preparation is not quick, but this decadent treat is worth your time. Do make sure to pop your can of coconut milk in the fridge the night before. Stored in an airtight container in the freezer, this will last up to 2 weeks.

Lime-juice tip: Whole foods are best, so try not to substitute bottled juice for fresh-squeezed.

Serves 6

Crust
- » 1 cup raw cashews
- » ½ cup unsweetened coconut flakes
- » 6 medjool dates, pitted
- » pinch sea salt

Filling
- » 3 ripe avocados, cut into chunks
- » 1 tbsp virgin coconut oil
- » juice of 5 limes (10 tbsp)
- » zest of 1 lime
- » ¼–⅓ cup maple syrup, to taste
- » 1 can full-fat coconut milk, refrigerated for a few hours or overnight

1. For the crust, in a food processor, grind the cashews and coconut flakes into a coarse meal. Add the pitted dates and a pinch of salt, and pulse until combined. Press evenly into the bottom of a springform pan or 9-inch pie plate and set aside.
2. For the filling, head back to your food processor or Vitamix. Toss in the avocados, coconut oil, lime juice and zest, and maple syrup. Blend until smooth and creamy, about 30 to 60 seconds.
3. Remove the coconut milk from the fridge, being sure not to shake it. Open the can and carefully scoop out the top thick coconut cream into a large bowl. Pour the avocado lime mixture into the bowl and stir lightly until combined.
4. Pour the filling onto the crust and spread evenly. Place in the freezer for 2 to 3 hours, or until the centre is firm. Slice, serve, and swoon.
5. On the off chance you have leftovers, put the tart back into the freezer. Pull it out and let it rest for 10 to 15 minutes so it'll be fork tender when you serve.

Vanilla Bean Chia Pudding

This dessert is so simple and delicious that you'll probably want to eat it for breakfast. We say, do it! When dessert is light and refreshing with the bonus of keeping your digestive system happy, you're actually encouraged to go back for seconds. Add variety with different Qi-moving fruits. Our favourite topper is stewed fresh spring rhubarb.

Prep tip: Make sure to leave time (at least 2 hours or, even better, overnight) for this to "set."

Serves 4

Pudding
- » 1 cup chia seeds
- » 4 cups almond (or soy) milk
- » 4 tbsp pure maple syrup (or honey)
- » Seeds from 1 vanilla bean (slice in half lengthwise, scrape out seeds) OR 2 tsp pure vanilla extract
- » pinch sea salt

Toppings
- » plum slices
- » raspberries
- » pink grapefruit wedges
- » peach slices
- » strawberries
- » stewed rhubarb

1. For the pudding, in a large bowl, combine all the ingredients and whisk thoroughly until well combined. Then whisk again to really ensure it's well combined. Cover and set aside on the kitchen counter for a minimum of 2 hours or overnight. Occasionally stir the pudding as it thickens.
2. When you're ready to serve, take out the vanilla pod, scoop into pretty glass bowls, and top with your choice of delicious fruit.

Yin Deficiency Reset

What's Happening in Your Body when Your Yin Is Deficient?

Pssst, hey you. Yes, you, the one who gets more done in a day than anyone else. The super-achiever who feels so good when others rave about your ability to tear through tasks at warp speed. You're whipping through life like a Tasmanian Devil, trailing a wake of (self) destruction. What could possibly go wrong?

Well, here's the deal: your pace is unsustainable. Your energy is sapped, zapped, and depleted. You've been running on fumes for a while now, probably years. Simply put, you're exhausted. You dream of finding that magical Fountain of Youth to keep you going, but you've tried everything and nothing has given you back your old pizzazz.

When Yin is deficient, your nervous system is strung out, leading to a typical pattern of symptoms.

Physical symptoms can be heat-like, such as low-grade fever, hot flashes, night sweats, hot hands and feet, a flushed face, and sore joints. You might also experience dryness such as a dry cough, dry mouth and throat, and a tendency to sip small amounts of fluid all day.

Emotionally and mentally, you may feel restless, easily agitated, frazzled, anxious, irritable, or on edge, with a tendency toward self-criticism and uneasiness.

Yin Deficiency can be described as adrenal fatigue, in which your batteries are deeply drained. You've got an abundance of false energy, making you feel simultaneously wired and tired. Ever stay up watching late-night TV even though you're utterly wiped out? That's a classic Yin-deficiency sign, and a red flag alerting you to begin nourishing and replenishing your Yin.

To understand Yin Deficiency, it helps to get your head around Yin and Yang, the complementary forces of nature at the core of Traditional Chinese Medicine (TCM). Very simply, Yang is active, light, and warm; it brings change. Yin is quiet, dark, and cool; it maintains stability.

Yin and Yang are constantly at play through all of nature. Take an egg and sperm, for example. The sperm remains true to Yang in its explosive, penetrating nature. The egg remains true to Yin, waiting patiently in a calm, controlled environment. Life begins when they come together to create a fertilized embryo.

Yin and Yang are not separate or static. They are constantly balancing and depending upon each other. We see this in the black and white Yin Yang symbol, where each is contained within the other amidst a swirl of movement.

Yin and Yang are active in our bodies as the sympathetic and parasympathetic nervous systems. You may not be familiar with these terms, but you know how they make you feel.

The sympathetic nervous system is Yang in nature; it responds to stimuli, gets you moving, and creates the fight-flight sensations that bombard you daily, keeping you addicted to a frenetic pace and overwork.

The parasympathetic nervous system is Yin in nature; it is responsible for your body's rest-and-digest function. You know, that feeling of "ahhhh" when you sink into the couch at the end of the day — that's your parasympathetic nervous system recovering and replenishing from the general overstimulation of your life. In other words, it's your Yin being nourished. It's the real-deal Fountain of Youth you've been looking for in all the wrong places.

What Yin Deficiency can look like

Ashley is 43 years old and can't remember how long she's been living on coffee and Red Bull. Her high-stress job in the financial industry keeps her on the go, and she's too restless to make time for self-care. Being busy makes her feel high, so she wants to go-go-go all day long. What's worse, at bedtime she hits a second wind that keeps her rolling well into the night.

Here are the signs that Ashley needs the Yin Deficiency Reset:

- Wired and tired (a key sign of Yin Deficiency)
- No idea how to relax
- Trouble falling asleep at night
- Night sweats
- Anxious, restless, and constantly self-critical

Estrogen, our most Yin hormone, nourishes and calms us. As Ashley is aging, she's producing less estrogen, putting her more at the mercy of her stress hormones. She's been working hard, with little rest, for a long time, and this has consumed a lot of her vital resources. Now, she's heading into perimenopause depleted.

Here's how Ashley will know the Yin Deficiency Reset is working:

- A lot more relaxed and at ease
- Able to fall asleep and have a deep, restful sleep
- Greater resilience to handle stress
- Decrease in overheating, night sweats, and hot flashes
- Energy feels good most of the time
- Can soak up the quiet without needing to keep her mind/hands busy with cell phone and constant busyness

Goals for Building Yin

Physically, nourished Yin carries fluids, nutrients, and vital messages throughout your whole body, keeping you grounded and fertile. Once replenished, Yin will constantly refill your well of reserve energy.

Emotionally and mentally, Yin shows up as inner calm, self-acceptance, and the ability to be deeply present to your life. Yin provides a still point, an anchor for all the activity of Yang in your days. Nourished Yin gives you the capacity to self-soothe and continuously restore your emotional and mental energy.

Your battery will be charged up with the goodness of whole, nourishing foods. No more running on fumes. Kiss false energy goodbye. You might not even return to your regular cuppa Joe because you've grown to love having energy that's steady, calm, and grounded.

Kitchen Medicine for Building Yin

We're going to get your kitchen set up with everything you need to heal from Yin Deficiency so you can feel replenished, at ease, and clear-minded. Here are your three key words to describe the foods that will help you rebuild Yin:

- Dark
- Watery
- Salty

Dark-coloured foods, like blackberries, black beans, and black sesame seeds, are powerhouse Yin builders.

Foods with a high water content will quench your thirst and cool down your body and mind. All fruits are nutrient dense and excellent for hydrating the body, but the best Yin builders are the watery ones, like melons, oranges, and dark-coloured berries. Veggies with a high water content, like water chestnuts and cucumbers, are especially thirst quenching and excellent for cooling down a hot, agitated mind and body.

Naturally salty foods, like pork, seaweed, fish, oysters, miso, and tamari soy sauce are also great Yin builders. Pork is our top meat choice for its health benefits. As for seafood, eating white fish has more of a cooling effect on the body than pink-fleshed fish like salmon. Seaweeds are highly therapeutic, so be sure to include them. An easy snack is a sheet of nori, the seaweed used for wrapping sushi. Enjoy its light crunchiness right out of the bag or get creative and wrap it around some leftover stir-fried veggies and rice and call it lunch. For a quick hit of mineral-rich coolness, toss some kelp (aka kombu) or seaweed salt into your soup or stock.

The name of the game for all of the Yin Yang Resets is eating whole foods. *But for building Yin, the QUALITY of your food is as important as WHAT you eat. The life force in your food is the ultimate healer, and that depends on HOW the food is grown.*

Yin deficient people need replenishing from the deepest source of nourishment, Mother Earth. So, join the slow food movement. Your Yin (and Momma Earth) will love you right back. Whenever you can, buy locally grown organic food and support artisans who select and combine ingredients with patience and care. Check out your local farmer's market. Scandalize the neighbours by planting raised beds in your front yard. No yard? See if there's any space in a community garden. Grow some greens on your patio or microgreens and herbs in a window.

Interestingly, eating dairy is encouraged for replenishing Yin (you're welcome!). Deeply nourishing and calming, milk from a mammal is the ultimate life-sustaining food for development and growth. Did you know that milk contains morphine-like proteins called casomorphins that have an opioid effect on the body? They induce a sense of calm, happiness, and relaxation, which is exactly what you need when you're Yin deficient. But don't overdo it. A small amount goes a long way and over-consumption can have the opposite effect. Buy the best-quality milk you can find, ideally from organic, grass-fed, happy animals.

NOT eating certain foods will also help you get your mojo back. Your body is already depleted and parched, so eating foods that burn up fluids will make your symptoms worse. This means avoid overeating foods that are hot and spicy, like mouth-burning chili peppers, cinnamon, and an excess of ginger.

Alcohol and stimulants like caffeine, cigarettes, and marijuana consume Yin quickly, so steer clear for now. If you love the taste of coffee, Dandy Blend is an excellent alternative. If you need a little bit of caffeine to help you through the transition, green tea will give you energy while cooling your body. (See "How and why to get off coffee" on page 36.)

Our goal is to help you become a Yin-building kitchen ninja, choosing and preparing nutrient-dense foods and tossing the crave-inducing processed junk that keeps you down. We want to make it easy for you to rebuild the deep energy reserves you need to move forward with your life.

Getting Started with building Yin

Your symptoms are the warning lights on the dashboard. Congratulations for having the self-love to stop and check your engine.

You might be a little annoyed with us, because we're going to encourage you to eliminate all the crutches that keep your false energy going during the day. You'll probably want to fight us and cheat on the reset. But you've landed here for a reason. Deep down, you know the way you've been living is not sustainable.

Yes, it's hard to give up being admired for your jaw-dropping ability to get shit done. But as your frazzled nerves get soothed and replenished by this diet, you'll start moving through your day with grounded energy and a youthful sense of ease. This will not only feel amazing, it may just inspire people around you to up their own self-care game. Instead of just impressing, you'll be sharing the love.

It's this simple: eat these slow, sustainably grown foods and feel better. Soon, you'll start to get the hang of picking Yin-building foods and even modifying your favourite recipes to include them. Let mother earth and your kitchen heal you.

Activities for Building Yin

Quick review: your Yin is depleted because you've been working too hard and depleting your physical resources. When it comes to exercise, your restless energy may be urging you to choose hot, sweaty, high-intensity movement, because that's the way you roll. You may even think exercise calms you down, but in your present state, vigorous exercise actually creates more burnout. You may want to move, but what you need is rest.

So, please, step away from that bootcamp. We encourage you to avoid strenuous exercise, at least until you rebuild your Yin. Instead, choose slow, peaceful activities like these and practice them with awareness:

- Yin and restorative yoga
- A saunter in the woods
- Swimming
- Gardening
- Snowshoeing (take it easy!)
- Meditation

Extra points for replacing bright lights and blue screens with candlelight after sundown!

Beverages for Building Yin

Daily green drink – 1 glass spirulina per day, following the serving size on the bottle

Herbal coffee – Dandy Blend (we love this coffee substitute)

Herbal hot and iced teas – See "How to make medicinal teas" on page 61. Traditional Medicinals have some great Yin-building teas:

- Nettle Leaf tea
- Burdock with Nettle Leaf tea
- Green Tea
- Peppermint
- Lemon Balm
- Hibiscus
- Mother's Milk Shatavari Cardamom (NOT just for moms, amazing for men and women)

Also try Tulsi (Holy Basil) from Organic India Tulsi Tea.

Yin Deficiency Reset Food Chart

Fruits	Vegetables	Grains
Bananas	Avocados	Amaranth
Blackberries	Beets	Barley
Blueberries	Bok choy	Kamut
Cantaloupe	Cauliflower	Millet
Goji berries	Cucumbers	Quinoa
Kiwis	Green beans	Rice
Melons	Leafy greens	Teff
Mulberries	Lettuce	**Herbs**
Oranges	Organic potatoes	
Organic grapes	Organic spinach	Cilantro
Organic pears	Organic tomatoes	Marjoram
Persimmons	Sprouts	Nettle
Raspberries	Water chestnuts	Peppermint
Watermelon	Zucchini	Sea salt

Organic Protein	Additional	Foods to Avoid
Black beans	All nuts: especially cashews and walnuts	Shrimp
Black soybeans		GMO foods
Clams	All seeds: especially black sesame seeds and hemp seeds	Spicy foods
Cow dairy		Red meat
Duck		Alcohol
Eggs	Butter	Lots of ginger
Goat dairy	Coconut milk	Coffee
Kidney beans	Duck fat	Non-organic foods
Lima beans	Extra virgin olive oil	
Mung beans	Organic gelatin	
Oysters	Organic soy milk	
Pork	Seaweed	
Sardines	Virgin coconut oil	
Soy/tofu		
White fish		

*Tip: No cigarettes or vaping

Sample Yin-Building Meal Plans

Day 1

Breakfast: Swiss Chard Bacon Frittata and a cup of Green Tea
Snack: Coconut yogurt with fresh berries and hemp seeds
Lunch: Deli Ham Avocado Wraps
Snack: Banana and cashew butter and a cup of Lemon Balm tea
Dinner: Basil Zucchini Quinoa Soup

Day 2

Breakfast: Basil Zucchini Quinoa Soup
Snack: Walnuts and seed mix with dried mulberries and goji berries and a cup of Green Tea
Lunch: Mung Bean Hummus Platter
Snack: Persimmon wedges with thinly sliced prosciutto
Dinner: Beet Risotto

More Snack Options

- Small bowl of red of black grapes
- Cup of bone broth
- Berries and diced kiwi with a squeeze of lime juice and a cup of Hibiscus Tea
- Organic pear and organic cheddar cheese slices

Day 3

Breakfast: Cacao Berry Smoothie and a cup of Green Tea
Snack: Sliced veggies and a hard boiled egg
Lunch: Beet Salad with Crumbled Goat Cheese & Black Sesame Seeds
Snack: Black Bean Brownie
Dinner: Fish Tacos

Day 4

Breakfast: Mulberry Walnut Banana Oatmeal and a cup of Nettle Leaf tea
Snack: Avocado slices wrapped with Roasted Seaweed Snacks
Lunch: Barley Mushroom Cucumber Salad
Snack: Miso soup with veggies & tofu
Dinner: Cilantro Mung Beans & Rice

More Snack Options

- Rice crackers with goat cheese
- Cantaloupe and watermelon slices with cashews
- Cauliflower, cherry tomatoes, and cucumbers with black bean hummus

Yin-Building Breakfasts

Cacao Berry Smoothie

This is a great quick breakfast or snack. But please remember that cold foods can put out your digestive "fire," so be sure to let this warm up to room temperature before drinking. (Get the full story on page 49 for using smoothies as part of your healing.) The good news? Chocolate for breakfast, yo!

Protein tip: We like Genuine Health Fermented organic vegan protein powder in this smoothie because the added stevia makes it extra delicious. But go ahead and use whatever protein powder you have on hand (see page 48 for more on protein options).

Chocolate lovers tip: For a rich, dark chocolate treat, add 1 tablespoon of cocoa powder (we love Camino) and reduce the cacao nibs to 1 tablespoon.

Serves 1

- ½ green tipped banana, broken into chunks
- ½ cup berries: blackberries, blueberries, raspberries
- 2 tbsp cacao nibs (we use Navitas Naturals)
- 1 cup almond (or soy or coconut) milk
- 1-2 cups water
- 1 tbsp hemp seeds
- 1 scoop protein powder

1. Toss all the ingredients into a blender or Vitamix and blend for about 30 seconds, until thoroughly combined.
2. Serve sprinkled with a few cacao nibs.

Mulberry Walnut Banana Oatmeal

Go ahead, sing it, you know you want to: "Here we go 'round the mulberry bush ..." Seriously, though, mulberries are so delicious, you'll want to munch on them as a snack, and we say DO IT. Packed with Yin-nourishing goodness, mulberries add a sweet depth to this classic dish. A patient of ours feeds them to her toddler grandson and now he asks for "nanaberries."

Protein tip: To boost your protein, pair with our Cacao Berry Smoothie on page 301.

Serves 2

Oats
- » 2 cups water
- » 1 cup uncooked rolled or quick oats

Toppings
- » 1 banana, sliced
- » ½ cup walnut halves
- » 4 tbsp dried mulberries (we use Navitas Naturals)
- » optional: almond/organic soy/coconut milk

1. In a medium saucepan, bring the water and oats to a boil, then turn down and simmer for about 5 minutes, stirring a few times. Adjust the liquid and cooking time to your liking (or according to package directions). Some people like their oats porridgey, while others like them al dente.
2. Serve topped with fruit and walnuts. Pour on a little bit of almond/soy/coconut milk, if you like.

Lemon Blueberry "Top of the Muffin to You!"

You know you only want the muffin top. Hey, we're not judging. With a nod to Seinfeld for keeping us entertained in the '90s, bake up a batch of these muffins, pull off the stump, and savour. The sour hit of lemon and sweet burst of blueberries will have you tucking them into your lunch for a healthy afternoon pick-me-up. Pair with a cup of lemon balm tea and chill out.

Protein tip: To boost your protein, pair with our Cacao Berry Smoothie, on page 301.

Makes 1 dozen

Dry
- 1½ cups teff flour (we use Bob's Red Mill)
- ½ cup tapioca flour
- 2 tsp baking powder
- ½ tsp baking soda
- 2 tbsp chia seeds (preferably black), ground in a coffee grinder or Vitamix

Wet
- 2 organic eggs, beaten
- 2 bananas, mashed
- 1 cup almond (or soy) milk
- ⅓ cup melted organic butter (or virgin coconut oil)
- ½ cup coconut palm (or organic) sugar
- zest of 1 organic lemon (top layer only, not bitter white underneath)
- 1 cup blueberries

1. Preheat the oven to 350°F. Grease a 12-cup muffin tin, or do as we do and line with paper cups.
2. In a medium bowl, combine the dry ingredients.
3. In a large bowl, beat together the eggs and mashed bananas, then stir in the milk, melted butter, sugar, and lemon zest.
4. Slowly add the dry ingredients to the wet, stirring after each addition. Fold in the blueberries.
5. Pour the batter into the prepared muffin tin. Bake for 30 minutes or until a knife inserted in the centre comes out clean. Cool on a wire rack before serving.

Swiss Chard Bacon Frittata

Breakfast for dinner or dinner for breakfast? Either way, welcome to Club Med-icine. It's worth skipping your local drive-thru for this frittata, which just begs to be eaten cold standing at the counter. Eggs, chard, and pork are super Yin-boosting foods, channeling your force within and calming your body and mind.

Serves 4-6

- » 2 slices organic bacon
- » 8 large organic eggs
- » sea salt and freshly ground black pepper, to taste
- » ½ cup chopped onion
- » 1 small sweet potato, halved lengthwise and thinly sliced
- » 4 cups chopped organic Swiss chard

1. Preheat the oven to 425°F.
2. In a large, oven-proof frying pan over low heat, cook the bacon until golden. Drain on a paper towel, allow to cool, and chop into small pieces.
3. Pour out about half of the bacon grease and leave a very thin layer covering the bottom of the pan.
4. In a medium bowl, beat the eggs with a pinch of salt and pepper.
5. Over medium heat, sauté the onion in the remaining bacon grease until soft and translucent. Add the sweet potato and cook until soft, about 10 minutes. Add the chard and toss around until it's wilted.

6. Turn the heat down to low-medium. Pour the egg mixture over the vegetables and sprinkle on the bacon evenly. Cook for 2 minutes without stirring.
7. Place the frying pan into the oven and bake for 20 to 30 minutes, until the frittata is puffy and set in the middle.
8. Slice into 6 pieces and serve with a mixed green salad.

Yin-Building Lunches

Beet Salad with Crumbled Goat Cheese & Black Sesame Seeds

Beets take some time to cook, BUT they're one of the most nourishing foods you can eat. We love having beets on hand, so why not cook up a large batch to sustain you through the week? The major yin producers here are black sesame seeds and goat cheese. The salad itself takes only a couple of minutes to prepare once you've got the beets ready, so it's a great recipe to keep on standby.

Serves 2

- » 3 medium-to-large beets
- » ½ tsp sea salt
- » 3 cups green beans, ends trimmed off
- » 2 tsp olive oil
- » 1-2 tsp balsamic vinegar
- » 4 tbsp soft organic goat cheese
- » 1 package alfalfa sprouts
- » 2 tsp black sesame seeds (white are fine, if you can't find black)
- » sea salt and freshly ground black pepper, to taste

1. Scrub the beets and put them into a pot large enough to cover them with water by 2 inches. Add the ½ tsp salt, bring to a boil, and cook for about 45 minutes, or until tender when pierced with a fork.
2. Meanwhile, steam the green beans for about 2 minutes, until bright green and still crunchy.

3. When the beets are cooked, drain them and let them cool. Once cool enough to handle, slip off the skins with a paper towel. Cut the beets into bite-sized chunks.
4. To serve, divide the beets and beans onto two plates and drizzle with the olive oil and balsamic vinegar. Crumble the goat cheese overtop and pile on a handful of alfalfa sprouts. Sprinkle with the sesame seeds and season with salt and pepper. Fast, nourishing, and delicious!

Deli Ham & Avocado Wraps

Ummm, yes please, I'd like to order a deli ham wrap. Oh wait, I'm the cook? No worries, this is so easy, I'll have it whipped up in minutes. Make these lunches to go for the rest of your crew knowing you'll be enjoying yours in peace and quiet, slow-food Yin style! Ham is one of the best meats to moisten dryness and calm your nerves, so pile it on and recharge your batteries.

Wrap tip: Try a variety of gluten-free wraps and find your favourite. We love coconut, cassava, almond flour and dehydrated veggie wraps for lunch. Find them at your local health food store (check in the frozen foods).

Serves 2

- » 2 almond flour tortilla wraps
- » 6 slices organic deli ham
- » mixed greens
- » 1 organic tomato, diced
- » 1 avocado, sliced
- » Dijon mustard

1. Preheat the oven to 350°F.
2. Pop the tortilla wraps in the oven and warm them for a minute or two, until they're soft and chewy (but not crisp).
3. Spread a little Dijon mustard on each wrap and top with 3 slices of ham, a handful of mixed greens, diced tomato, and sliced avocado.
4. Wrap up and enjoy your quick-and-easy lunch.

Barley Mushroom Cucumber Salad

Say so long to night sweats and fiery sensations that heat up your days. You'll be cool as a cucumber with this salad. Allow the flavours to mingle by tossing it together at the beginning of the week, and have on hand for a quick lunch or as a side dish with grilled fish.

Serves 4

Salad
- 1 cup barley (or quinoa for a gluten-free option), rinsed
- 1 tbsp olive oil
- 5 cups sliced button mushrooms
- 2 carrots, grated
- 2 green onions, thinly sliced
- 1 cup diced cucumber
- ¼ cup minced cilantro

Dressing
- 2 tbsp tamari soy sauce (or Bragg Liquid Aminos)
- 1 tbsp sesame oil
- 1 tbsp apple cider vinegar
- freshly ground black pepper, to taste

1. In a medium saucepan, cook the barley with 3 cups of water for 45 to 60 minutes. Drain and set aside.
2. In a large frying pan, heat the olive oil over medium heat. Sauté the mushrooms until soft and most of the liquid has evaporated. Set aside.

3. While the mushrooms cook, combine all the dressing ingredients in a small bowl.
4. In a medium bowl, combine the cooked barley and mushrooms with the carrots, green onions, cucumber, and cilantro. Drizzle with the dressing, grind in a little pepper, and you're all set to cool that fire.

Mung Bean Hummus Platter

Satisfy your inner snacker with this hummus and crudités combo. The pulse and power of this dish lies in the medicinal properties of the mung beans. These amazing little guys are able to detox and cool that deep-burning fire and nourish you from the inside out.

Batch tip: While you're at it, whip up a double batch of hummus so you'll have enough for making the Black Bean Burgers (coming up in the dinners).

Serves 4

Hummus
- ½ cup dried mung beans, rinsed
- 1½ cups water
- ¼ cup tahini (sesame seed paste)
- 1 garlic clove, minced
- ½ cup water
- ½–1 tsp sea salt
- juice of ½ lemon

Serving options
- organic celery sticks
- carrot sticks
- organic sweet bell peppers
- cucumber slices
- black olives
- gluten-free crackers (Mary's Gone Crackers are a favourite)

1. Bring the mung beans to a boil in a medium saucepan with the 1½ cups of water. Reduce the heat and simmer, covered, for 45 to 60 minutes, until beans are tender. If the beans are drying out before they're cooked, add a bit more water. If you've got water left at the end, drain it off.
2. In a food processor, combine the cooked beans with the tahini, garlic, water, salt, and lemon juice, and blend until smooth and creamy. If the mixture is too thick, add a little more water.
3. Serve in a bowl with an assortment of fresh vegetables and gluten-free crackers.

Yin-Building Dinners

Sautéed Portobellos with Crumbled Goat Cheese & Millet

Who needs a plate when you have a portobello mushroom? Well, ok, you still do. But, portobellos make great vessels for all those Yin-nourishing foods such as millet, goat cheese, butter, and bok choy. This scrumptious dinner is a cinch to prepare if you have some cooked millet on hand. And why not eat more millet? This quick-cooking, gluten-free grain cooks up light and fluffy in a jiff, and you can substitute it for rice in many recipes.

Protein tip: To boost your protein, sauté up a side of organic firm tofu or tempeh.

Serves 4

- 2 cups millet
- 4 cups vegetable stock
- 1 tsp organic butter
- 1 tbsp olive oil
- 4 portobello mushrooms, stems removed, caps wiped clean
- ½ red onion, sliced into rings and separated
- 1 organic yellow bell pepper, sliced into rings
- pinch sea salt and freshly ground black pepper
- 6 cups baby bok choy, chopped into large pieces
- 4 tbsp organic goat cheese

1. In a medium saucepan, cook the millet in the stock for about 15 to 20 minutes, or until all the liquid is

absorbed. Have a bit more stock on hand to add if the grains dry out before they're soft.
2. In a medium frying pan, heat the butter and olive oil over medium heat and toss in the mushroom caps. Cover with a lid and cook for about 10 minutes.
3. Add the onion and pepper rings, season with salt and pepper, and cook, stirring occasionally, for an additional 10 minutes, or until all the veg is tender and juicy.
4. Meanwhile, steam the bok choy in a steamer basket for 2 to 3 minutes.
5. To serve, place the mushroom cap top side down and scoop some millet on top. Top with sautéed veggies, a tablespoon of crumbled goat cheese, and the steamed bok choy on the side.

Fish Tacos

We always order the fish tacos when we're at a restaurant. They're just such a treat. Well, we're pretty excited that now we can chow down on this fave right at home. White fish, avocado, tomatoes, and sprouts are excellent Yin builders, so these are not only tasty and easy to prepare, they're healing too.

Taco tip: You can use either fresh or frozen corn tacos, usually found in the refrigerator or freezer section of your health food store. If you can't find corn tortillas, substitute cassava, almond flour, rice, or dehydrated veggie wraps.

Serves 4

Fish
- » 1 lb firm white fish fillets
- » juice from ½ lime
- » sea salt and freshly ground black pepper, to taste

Avocado salsa
- » 1 avocado, diced
- » 2 tbsp finely diced organic sweet bell pepper
- » 2 tbsp finely diced red onion
- » juice from ½ lime

Tomato salsa
- » 2 medium organic tomatoes, diced
- » 1 tsp olive oil
- » ¼ cup minced cilantro

- » 2 tbsp olive oil
- » soft organic corn tortillas
- » 1 package alfalfa sprouts

1. Place the fillets in a shallow dish (like a pie plate), squeeze the lime juice over top, and sprinkle with salt and pepper. Marinate in the fridge for about 20 minutes.
2. Meanwhile, make the salsas in two small mixing bowls.
3. In bowl #1, combine the avocado salsa ingredients with a pinch of salt and pepper.
4. In bowl #2, combine the tomato salsa ingredients with another pinch of salt and pepper.
5. Preheat the oven to 400°F.
6. Heat the 2 tbsp of olive oil over medium heat in a frying pan. Cook the fish for about 3 minutes on each side, or until done to your liking.
7. Heat the corn tortillas in the oven for 1 to 2 minutes, until warm but still soft.
8. To serve, spoon fish into the centre of each tortilla and top with the salsas and a handful of alfalfa sprouts. Taco heaven!

Basil Zucchini Quinoa Soup

Got leftovers? Those veggies hiding in the back of your fridge are begging to heal you. The real flavour factor in this dish is the fresh basil, so go ahead and be generous. This is a dish you'll want to go back to for seconds. Zucchini and quinoa are certified top-notch Yin builders. Adding them to a hydrating soup base will amplify their healing credentials.

Garnish tip: Try topping your soup with a dollop of organic sour cream or yogurt to really boost its Yin-nourishing properties. Or, if you're dairy free, pan fry some organic tempeh and crumble on top for a protein boost.

Serves 4

- ½ cup diced onion
- 2 tbsp olive oil
- 8 cups vegetable broth
- 3 cups peeled and diced sweet potatoes
- ¾ cup quinoa, rinsed
- 1 cup diced organic zucchini
- 1 bunch organic kale, stems removed, leaves finely chopped
- 1 tbsp or more finely chopped fresh basil (or 1 tsp dried)

1. In a large pot, sauté the onion in the olive oil over medium heat until soft (about 5 minutes).
2. Add your broth, sweet potatoes, and quinoa and bring to a boil. Reduce the heat and cook for 20 minutes, until the quinoa looks plump and cooked.
3. Add the zucchini and kale (and dried basil, if using) and cook for another 10 minutes. Stir in the fresh basil and remove from the heat and serve.

Cilantro Mung Beans & Rice

We love 3-for-1 meals around here: breakfast, lunch, and dinner is served. If mung beans came in a can, this dish would be even easier but, alas, these little babies need cooking. Say so long to all-day heat waves in your body. This curative dish will cool your overheated body with every bite.

Serves 4

- » 1 cup dried mung beans
- » 3 cups water
- » 2 cups brown rice (we like basmati or short grain)
- » 4 cups water
- » 1 tbsp olive oil
- » 1 small onion, diced
- » 1 large organic zucchini, quartered lengthwise and roughly chopped (about 2 cups)
- » 1-2 carrots, grated
- » 1½ tbsp tamari soy sauce (or Bragg Liquid Aminos)
- » ½ cup minced cilantro

1. Rinse the mung beans and bring them to a boil in a medium saucepan with 3 cups of water. Turn the heat down and simmer on low until done, about 45 to 60 minutes.
2. Meanwhile, in another medium saucepan, bring the rice to a boil with 4 cups of water. Turn the heat down and simmer on low until done, about 45 to 60

minutes. Add a bit more water if the grains dry out before they are cooked.
3. In a large frying pan, heat the olive oil over medium heat and sauté the onion until soft and translucent. Add the zucchini and carrots, and cook for about 5 minutes, until crisp-tender.
4. Add the cooked mung beans to the pan along with the tamari or Bragg's and cilantro, and combine well. Remove from heat.
5. To serve, put a large scoop of hot rice on a plate and heap with the veggies and beans.

Black Bean Burgers

We're all about harnessing the superpower of leftovers to make meal prep a breeze. If you whipped up extra Mung Bean Hummus (page 314), you'll have these burgers plated in no time. Invite the neighbours over. You don't have to mention the healing power of food, just say "it's burger time!"

Bread crumb tip: If you don't have gluten-free bread crumbs on hand, you can grind toasted or stale slices of gluten-free bread in your food processor.

Lighten-up tip: Eat the burger patty in a crunchy lettuce leaf for a lighter meal. Serve with lots of sauteed veggies on the side.

Serves 4

Burgers
- 14-oz can organic black beans, rinsed and drained
- ½ cup diced organic green pepper
- 1 clove garlic, minced (optional)
- ¼ cup hummus (hello, leftovers!)
- 1 organic egg, beaten
- ¼ cup minced cilantro
- ¾ tsp sea salt
- freshly ground black pepper, to taste
- ½-¾ cup gluten-free bread crumbs (2 piece of gluten free bread)
- olive oil for frying

For serving (feel free to get creative)
- 4 gluten-free buns
- organic tomato slices
- sautéed veggies (organic zucchini, sweet bell peppers, Swiss chard, etc.)
- alfalfa sprouts
- cucumber slices
- avocado slices
- organic mayonnaise (Veganaise is our favourite)

1. In a medium bowl, mash up the black beans with a potato masher or chop roughly in a food processor (but leave it chunky). Stir in the green pepper, garlic, hummus, egg, cilantro, salt, and pepper until well combined.
2. Mix in enough bread crumbs to make patties that hold together and are not too sticky. You may need a little more or less. Form into 4 burger-sized patties.
3. Heat 1 tbsp of olive oil in a frying pan over medium heat and cook the patties until they are golden, about 3 to 4 minutes on each side.
4. Serve on a toasted gluten-free bun with any or all of the toppings.

Stuffed Acorn Squash

Raise your hand if you love a good night's sleep. We thought so. This nourishing dish has the healing properties to help cool that inner fire so you'll wake rested in the morning. Watch out, night sweats and troubled sleep, because greens, millet, and squash are coming for you!

Serves 4

- 1 cup vegetable broth
- ½ cup millet
- 2 tbsp olive oil
- 1 onion, diced
- 1 organic sweet red bell pepper, diced
- ½ cup sliced button mushrooms
- 3 cups chopped collard greens
- ½ tsp dried sage
- ½ tsp sea salt
- freshly ground black pepper, to taste
- 2 acorn squash (about 1 lb each)
- ¼ cup pumpkin seeds

1. In a small saucepan, bring the broth and millet to a boil. Reduce heat to a low simmer and cook, covered, for about 15 to 20 minutes, until all the liquid is absorbed. Remove from the heat, fluff with a fork, and set aside.
2. Meanwhile, heat the olive oil in a large frying pan over medium heat, and sauté the onion until soft and translucent. Add the pepper and mushrooms,

and cook until soft. Add the chopped collard greens, sprinkle with sage, salt, and pepper, and cook until the greens are tender (up to 15 minutes for more mature collards).
3. Preheat the oven to 400°F.
4. Add the cooked millet to the vegetable mixture and stir until combined. Stir in the pumpkin seeds.
5. Cut each acorn squash in half, scoop out the seeds, and place on a baking sheet or in a casserole dish. Drizzle each half with a little bit of olive oil, stuff with the millet and vegetable mixture, and cover with foil.
6. Bake for 60 to 80 minutes, until the squash is fork tender. Remove the foil about 10 minutes before the end of baking to brown the filling a bit.

Beet Risotto

Yell "PINK RICE is ready" and watch as curious faces rock up to your table. Beets truly take on the pulse of the earth, with their long, penetrating roots gathering all the nutrients you need to heal. This one-dish wonder is sure to spark a deeply rooted love of self on your healing journey. We like to serve this alongside a heap of steamed green beans.

Serves 4

- 2 medium-large beets
- 1 small onion, diced
- 2 tbsp olive oil
- 1½ cups Arborio rice
- 4½ cups organic chicken (or vegetable) broth
- 2 tbsp organic butter
- ¼ cup grated organic Parmesan cheese (or old white cheddar)
- freshly ground black pepper, to taste

1. Place the beets in a medium saucepan with water to cover. Bring to a lively boil and cook for about 45 minutes, until fork tender. You may need to add more water as it evaporates. Drain and let cool. Use a paper towel to peel off the skins (it's fast, easy, and clean). Chop into 1-inch cubes.
2. In a large pot, sauté the onion in olive oil over medium heat until soft, making sure not to brown.

3. Stir in the Arborio rice and begin adding broth, ½ cup at a time, slowly stirring after each addition until it's almost absorbed.
4. When the broth is all added and absorbed, stir in the chopped beets, butter, cheese, and pepper. Combine well and serve piping hot and pink!

Yin-Building Desserts

Delicious Black Bean Brownies

OMG CHOCOLATE!!! You can confidently show up to your next dinner party rockin' brownies. Once everyone is hooked, you can drop the bomb that they're actually healthy because they're made with black beans. We had to "retest" this recipe a few times because the brownies kept disappearing – into our bellies – and we couldn't get out the door with a full pan!

Salt tip: If using unsalted butter or virgin coconut oil, add ¼ tsp sea salt to the recipe.

Makes an 8 by 8-inch pan

- » 14-oz can organic black beans, drained and rinsed
- » 2 organic eggs, beaten
- » 3 tbsp melted organic butter (or virgin coconut oil)
- » ½ cup coconut palm (or organic) sugar
- » ½ cup unsweetened cocoa powder
- » ½ tsp baking powder
- » 1 tsp pure vanilla extract

1. Preheat the oven to 350°F. Grease an 8 by 8-inch baking pan with butter or coconut oil.
2. Blend all ingredients in a food processor or Vitamix until mixture is smooth. Be sure there are no chunks of black beans or it won't taste right.
3. Pour the brownie mixture into the prepared baking pan, spreading evenly. Don't worry if it doesn't look like enough, as it will puff up a bit while cooking. Bake for 25 minutes.

4. Allow to cool before eating, as the brownies will be quite crumbly while hot.

Caramelized Bananas with Raspberries

Hot caramelized bananas, anyone? Umm, yes please. Satisfy your sweet tooth while replenishing your body's radiance with this sumptuously healthy dessert. Have this a few nights a week as a special treat. You not only deserve it, you owe it to yourself.

Serves 2

- » 3 tbsp organic butter
- » 3 tbsp coconut palm sugar (or organic sugar)
- » 1 banana, sliced in half lengthwise
- » ½ tsp pure vanilla extract
- » organic vanilla yogurt
- » small container fresh raspberries

1. In a medium frying pan, melt the butter and sugar together over medium-high heat. Add the banana halves and cook, stirring, for about 3 minutes or until bubbly and caramelized.
2. Pour in the vanilla and stir for another 30 seconds. Take off the heat.
3. To serve, fill small bowls with yogurt and pour the hot banana and caramel sauce on top. Sprinkle on some fresh raspberries and indulge.

Frequently Asked Questions

You might be wondering …

Can I really do this? It feels like a LOT and I'm not sure I have the time.

Yes, you can! We get it, though. You're worried about how you're going to pull this off while keeping the rest of your life on track. The great news is that restoring your own vital energy will make everything in your life feel more manageable. Setting realistic goals is your first step to positive change. This is not an all-or-nothing diet. Small steps are often the most powerful, so get real about what feels doable right now.

How about choosing just 1 to 3 recipes for the week? Pick the ones that sound the most delicious to you and try them out. If you don't like (or can't find) certain ingredients, change them up with foods from your Reset's food chart.

If this style of cooking and planning is new to you, give yourself lots of time and do NOT aim for perfection. Just keep making an effort, and you'll naturally become more present and mindful of what you're putting on the table and into your body.

Will I have to stay on the Yin Yang Reset forever?

No, these Resets are designed for short-term use, to balance and heal your current symptoms. Most people stay on them for 2 to 4 weeks. We suggest you check in after two weeks and redo the quiz to track your progress (page 21).

If your symptoms persist, continue for another two weeks. Some people stay on their Reset for up to three months (especially the Reset for Dampness, which can be more stubborn to shift).

If new symptoms show up, take the quiz again to help you determine which Reset is best for you now.

For maximum benefit, we strongly suggest working with an acupuncturist or Traditional Chinese Medicine practitioner as you do the Yin Yang Reset.

What if I can't find some of the ingredients?

You can always substitute with similar foods from the food chart for your Reset. You'll also find lots of alternatives suggested in the recipes. If you're determined to use a food you can't find locally, try shopping online (hello, Amazon).

Do I really have to give up coffee?

Yes, we encourage you to do your best to eliminate coffee, or at the very least substitute it with something like caffeine-free Dandy Blend, a herbal coffee substitute. What's so important about giving coffee a rest? You'll no longer be covering up your low energy with a stimulant. Now, you'll be able to bring your depleted energy back up naturally with foods, rather than a caffeine fix. As a transition, try green tea. It contains caffeine, but it's less taxing on your system and has added antioxidants. (See How and why to give up coffee, on page 36.)

I'm vegetarian / vegan / celiac / dairy-free / egg-sensitive, etc. Can I still use the recipes?

Yes, use your Reset's food chart as your ultimate guide and modify the recipes to fit your needs. Get creative by using your own recipes and subbing in food-chart ingredients where you can. The more you use the recipes, the better you'll get at improvising healing meals. As long as you're using ingredients from your Reset's food chart, you'll be healing your symptoms.

Can I do this diet while I'm pregnant?

Yes, but we have two main recommendations.

First, make sure you're consuming enough calories. Do not eliminate nuts, seeds, and fats, as these foods will help meet the caloric levels you need to grow a new life.

And second, avoid the daily green drinks (spirulina, chlorella, wheatgrass), as greens can have a detox effect, and you don't want toxins flooding into your bloodstream while you're pregnant.

The great news is that eliminating processed foods and all sources of gluten and dairy will radically benefit your gut and overall health, and the health of your growing baby. Please consult your family physician and an acupuncturist or Traditional Chinese Medicine practitioner to help guide you through dietary changes.

Can I do the Yin Yang Diet while I'm breastfeeding?

Yes, food is one of the safest forms of medicine and a great way to influence the health of both you and your baby.

Our main suggestion is that you maintain an adequate caloric intake. This is as important when you're breastfeeding as it was during pregnancy. Healthy fats are also essential to a baby's brain development, so make sure you keep foods in your diet that contain good fats.

Please also consult your family physician and an acupuncturist or Traditional Chinese Medicine practitioner to help guide you through dietary changes.

Can my child eat these meals with me?

Absolutely! Many of our recipes are kid tested. Children are surrounded by processed foods, so they'll benefit hugely from these nourishing alternatives.

Remember, though, this is YOUR reset, not theirs. Be respectful of their routine and keep serving them their regular foods alongside the Ying Yang recipes. When we're following one of the Resets, we eat one of the dinner recipes with the whole family, but we still serve our kids their regular breakfast, lunch, and snacks.

If you do make changes to your child's diet, make sure their caloric needs are still being met. They're growing like weeds, and they need energy.

Find ways to nurture a love for healthy foods while your kids are young. Involve them in shopping and meal prep when you have time. They'll learn valuable life skills and feel a sense of ownership over what's on their plate.

Get them hooked on whole foods now, and they'll thank you in the end – with their glowing good health!

When and how fast should I start the diet?

The key is to set yourself up for success. We find it's best not to start on a major holiday, birthday, vacation, or any other celebration that's likely to tempt you to "cheat."

Diving in with both feet is great, but you can also take a slow approach. Even changing 20 percent of your meals will help reduce symptoms.

However, to be rewarded with the deepest health transformation, you'll need to eventually take on 100 percent of the program.

I'm spending a lot of time cooking, is this normal?

Yes, when you first change your diet, you'll spend more time prepping and cooking. Yin Yang Reset is based on traditional Chinese herbal medicine, which uses food as medicine. Remind yourself that you're not just cooking, you're replacing all those bottles of pills with personalized therapeutic food formulas.

Your results will be worth the extra time. Have faith in yourself as you work these new kitchen practices into your routine. Change takes courage and self-love. We know you can do it!

What is the gut-brain connection and why does it matter?

Your gut and brain are intimate partners, rather like Yin and Yang. They are constantly sending physical and chemical signals to each other in what's called the gut-brain axis. Your brain and gut have a constant and direct effect on each other — and the rest of your body, too.

Until recently, conditions in the brain, like depression and anxiety, were thought to trigger conditions in the gut like IBS, Crohn's, pain, and bloating. But current thinking says it may be the other way around: trouble in the gut disrupts the brain, triggering mood changes.

This intimate gut-brain connection is why healing your gut can go such a long way toward clearing up "brain issues" like brain fog and anxiety. In fact, the gut is now called the second brain or enteric nervous system, the first brain being the central nervous system.

When you're not feeding your body foods that nourish, or you're eating in a stressed and hurried state, your gut sends hurtful messages to the brain that can cause inflammation throughout the body.

But by eating specific foods that rebalance your current symptoms, your gut begins to heal, which in turn heals your brain. Incorporating some of our lifestyle suggestions, such as exercise and meditation, will further heal your brain, which in turn circles back to heal your gut.

Yin Yang Reset helps your gut and brain support each other and brings you back into whole-body-and-mind harmony.

Throughout all of our meal plans you'll find the tools you need to rebuild a balanced system from brain to gut right down to your toes.

If a food isn't listed on my Reset's food chart, can I still eat it?

Go right ahead, as long as that food is not on your "avoid" list. To get your absolute best results, make sure most of your foods are from the food chart. Eat any other foods only in moderation.

Acknowledgments

Tara: This book was born from a challenging time in my life, the newborn days of my oldest son. Sleep deprived with a colicky baby had me feeling anxious with insomnia. My baby was finally starting to sleep during the night, but there I was, bug-eyed and staring at the ceiling, on high alert listening for my baby to wake up, even as he slept soundly.

I took some herbs for my insomnia, but they made my symptoms ten times worse. This left me feeling not only more anxious, but now I was afraid to take herbs again. That's when I turned to food as a safe and gentle solution. Well, the solution turned out to be far from gentle. Within three days of using food as medicine, the Traditional Chinese Medicine way, I started feeling remarkably better. After a month, I felt like myself again.

This book exists thanks to the encouragement of my late husband, Kelyn, who told me I should create a cookbook and share this wisdom with the masses. Kelyn is a silent creator of the Yin Yang Reset; he spent hours, months, and years listening to Sara and I pitch ideas, write and rewrite book drafts, and create social media posts and videos. He tasted recipes, made marketing suggestions, and helped us when we felt defeated, stuck, or without direction.

He was my biggest cheerleader, genuinely passionate about me pursuing soul-driven endeavours in my life.

Babe, thank you for supporting me in everything my heart set out to do, even when I was afraid to do it. And yes, I give you full credit for the name Yin Yang, as it spontaneously came to you on a drive home from the organic market one morning. Thank you for everything. I miss and love you so much.

Partnership means everything to me, and Sara is the most wonderful partner I could ever wish for. We came together seeking support as acupuncturists, moms, and creatives. Our meeting was a gift from the heavens. When I'm stuck, her creativity is free flowing. When I need a boost, she knows exactly what to say. When we both feel burned out, we kick back together, put the world on hold, and share a day of delicious meals, spa treatments, and indulgences that renew our spirit. Thank you for being my best friend, my rock, and my inspiration.

Sara: Writing a cookbook is a big job, but combine it with revamping outdated, and often confusing, Traditional Chinese Medicine food practices, and you've got double trouble. That's why this book had to be a team effort. Bringing it to print has taken us eight years, all thanks to the team of badass women we've had the pleasure of working with.

Tara, my ride or die. Without you hauling me to the edge, asking me to jump into a world of the unknown, we wouldn't be here today. To the countless hours of long-distance calls, our aging blue-lit faces, those big ugly tears, broken hearts, and full on belly laughs. I'd be lost without you. You are the shining light that brought this to fruition. Thank you for being brave every day.

I'm forever grateful to our co-author, Marial Shea. The way you make our words come to life with our sassy undertone and hilarity will always be pure magic in my eyes. Your patience, knowledge, infuriating clarity questions, dedication to this eight-year long project, and your friendship are sacred things. On the one hand, we want to sing your praises to the masses, but on the other hand, we don't want to share you!

To my boys who, for the sake of this book, have suffered through far too many – well, let's be polite and call them "meals." And given my undying love for cookbooks, you can bet there will be many more to come. Thank you for being patient with me as I rip through the kitchen like a hot mess of a tornado. I'm sorry for some of the things I made you eat, and I always appreciate your honesty. I owe you big time. Your love and unwavering support in this pursuit of my passion has made for a wild ride. There are no two other people I'd want to be riding this wave with.

To my parents, inlaws, and family, who literally have no idea what I do on the daily, but still support me every step of the way, thank you.

And to my spirit guides who have passed on the torch – my big brother Jason, Wade, Kelyn, and Grandma – this book is for you. I'll see your guidance and raise you a bestseller.

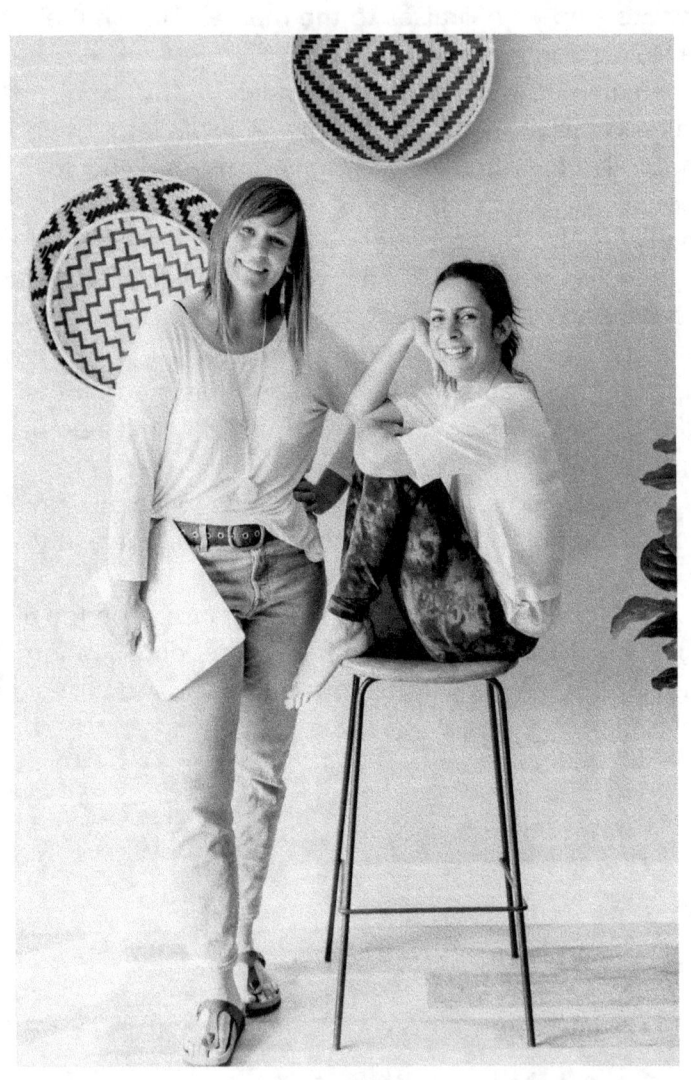

About the Authors

Tara Akuna, R.Ac, is a mother, entrepreneur, author, and acupuncturist living with her partner and children near Toronto, Canada. As a child, Tara watched her grandmother heal her breast cancer with a macrobiotic diet. She wished for bologna sandwiches and fruit gummies in her school lunches, but she's grateful she got miso soup, brown rice, and veggies instead. Today, kitchen medicine is the foundation of Tara's clinical practice as an acupuncturist.

Sara Ward, R.Ac, is a dedicated hockey mom living in Vancouver with her husband and son. She is a multi-passionate entrepreneur, author, acupuncturist, and founder of The Village Community clinic. During a health scare in her early twenties, when she was diagnosed with celiac disease, Sara fell deeply in love with using food as medicine. In her clinical practice, Sara's go to for everything is gut health. Every day at home, she practices what she preaches in the kitchen.

www.ingramcontent.com/pod-product-compliance
Lightning Source LLC
Chambersburg PA
CBHW071332080526
44587CB00017B/2807